Juice Your Mood

Flavor, Feelings, and Fun in Every Sip

Go ahead. Turn the page.

Juice Your Mood

Flavor, Feelings, and Fun in Every Sip

By

Monique L. Webb

MONKEY STUCK ADVENTURES

STORIES THAT STICK WITH YOU

Photography by Monique L. Webb

Published by Monkey Stuck Adventures LLC
Printed in the United States of America

First edition, 2025

Juice Your Mood
is dedicated to anyone who's
ever needed a reason
to feel better—
one sip at a time.

What's Inside

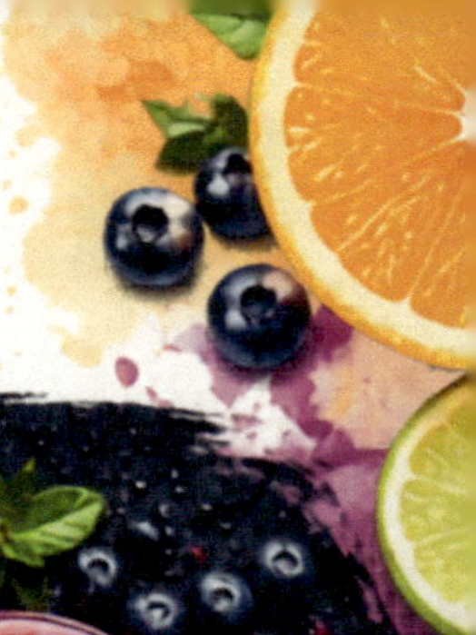

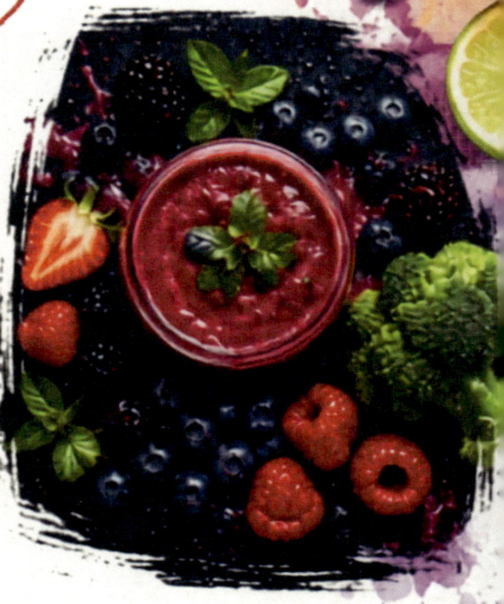

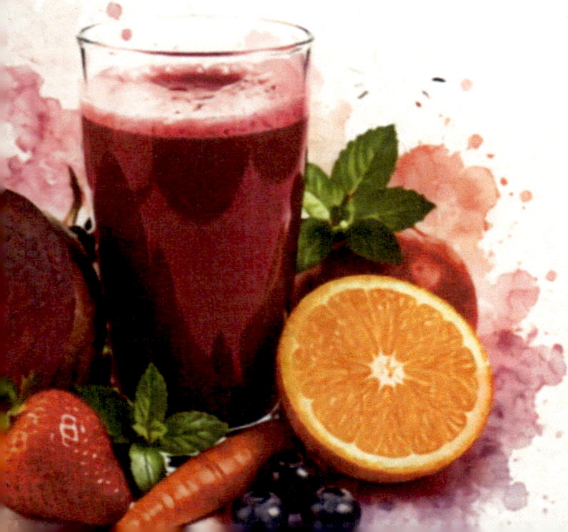

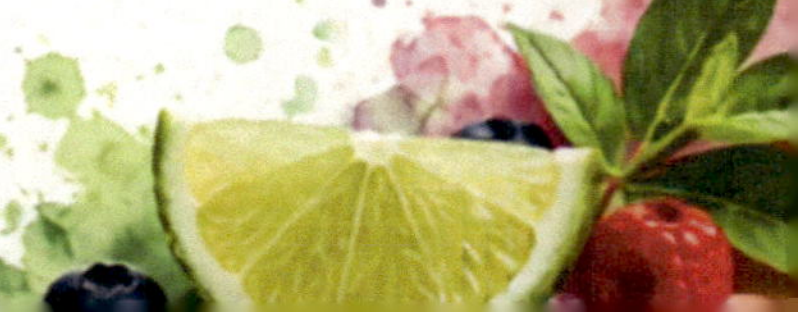

Every mood has a *flavor.*

Why this Book?

JUICE YOUR MOOD was created to make wellness feel fun. It's not meant to be intimidating; it's joyful, colorful, and full of personality.

This book doesn't judge you for how you feel. It simply says, **"Cool. Let's make something delicious for that."**

IT'S FOR the days you're energized, the days you're overwhelmed, and the days you're not sure what you're feeling at all. It's for anyone who's ever needed a tiny boost, a bright moment, or a reason to smile.

THE WHY? To help you sip your way through every mood, with flavor, feelings, and fun in every glass.

How it *Works*

Juice Your Mood is designed to meet you where you are, emotionally, physically, and realistically. You can read it straight through, or however you prefer. There's no wrong place to start.

Each juice is grouped by mood, represented by color. The moods/colors in this book are guides, not limits.

- Green — grounding, balance, leafy support
- Yellow / Orange — brightness, energy, clarity
- Red — nourishment, strength, deep support
- Purple — calm, reflection, brain-friendly blends
- Mixed Mood — complex days that don't fit neatly into one feeling

Before choosing a juice, you can ask yourself:

- How do I feel right now?
- What does my body want more of?
- What kind of support sounds good today?

Then flip to that mood and choose what speaks to you. You don't have to stay in one mood, and you don't have to feel the same tomorrow. That's the point. If you're unsure how you feel, there's probably a juice for that, too.

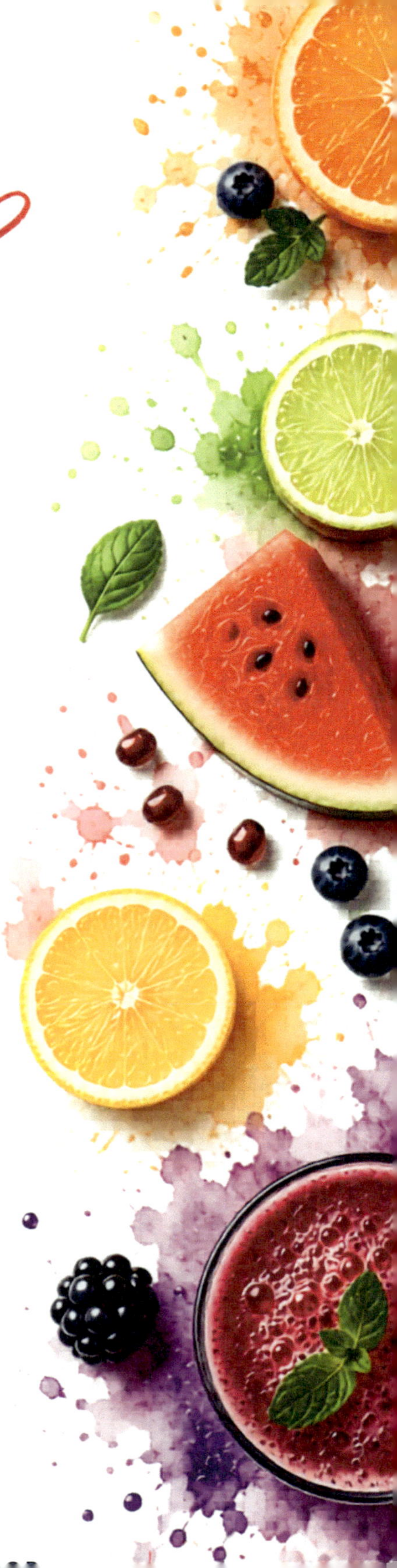

Housekeeping *Tips*

Dirty fruit and veggies will make your juice crunchy and not in a fun way. Wash your hands, produce, and juicer thoroughly.

Drink juices fresh as soon as possible. You decide. Refrigerate, if necessary. Do not drink spoiled juice.

Stir or shake juices if separation occurs; that's normal.

Follow the recipe as written. **DO NOT USE INGREDIENTS YOU ARE ALLERGIC TO OR SENSITIVE TO.** Substitute freely. Once you're familiar with it, you may find you want more or less of something. Each recipe makes one generous serving; adjust with water as needed, especially for thicker juices.

Some berry-based juices have a velvety, smooth texture—more like a thin smoothie than a traditional juice. That's normal and delicious.

When fresh fruit and vegetables aren't available, use frozen. Thaw before juicing.

Strain juices when you want less or no pulp. I use a nut milk bag.

A foam mustache is okay. Crunchy juice is not.

When in doubt, peel it. Remove pits. Juice greens before fruit.

Centrifugal (fast) and masticating (slow) juicers are effective. Yield may vary slightly depending on produce size, ripeness, and juicer efficiency.

Don't have a juicer? Use a blender, then strain through a fine mesh strainer, cheesecloth, or nut milk bag to remove the pulp.

Clean your machine shortly afterward. It makes life easier.

Use your juicer or blender according to the manufacturer's instructions.

Warning: Checking in with yourself might lead to accidentally taking care of yourself.

JUST OPENING THIS BOOK SHOWS YOU'RE IN THE MOOD TO JUICE. ♡

Top 5 *Mood* Favorites

When you need cozy and sweet

Chilling Cherry (p. 20)

Deep cherries, pears, and cinnamon comfort in a glass.

When you're ready to own the room

Purple Reign (p. 38)

Black grapes, blueberries, pomegranate seed, and lime.

When you're feeling salty and need to lean into it

Salty (p. 56)

Celery, cucumber, grapes, green apple, and lemon with crisp attitude.

When you need a punch of sunshine

Orange Sucker Punch (p. 64)

Orange, pineapple, lemon, and ginger with a bold citrus kick.

When life feels unhinged, but you're still going

Sweet Cheeks (p. 80)

Peaches, golden apple, pineapple, pear, lemon and ginger (optional).

Warning:

Do not use ingredients you are allergic or sensitive to. Always listen to your body and substitute ingredients as needed.

You can't pour from an *empty glass.*

So fill yours first.
With juice, obviously.

The moods are loading.

Juice Your Mood

Flavor, Feelings, and
Fun
in Every Sip

The *moods* are *loaded.*

Red Moods

Bold, grounding, and emotionally supportive

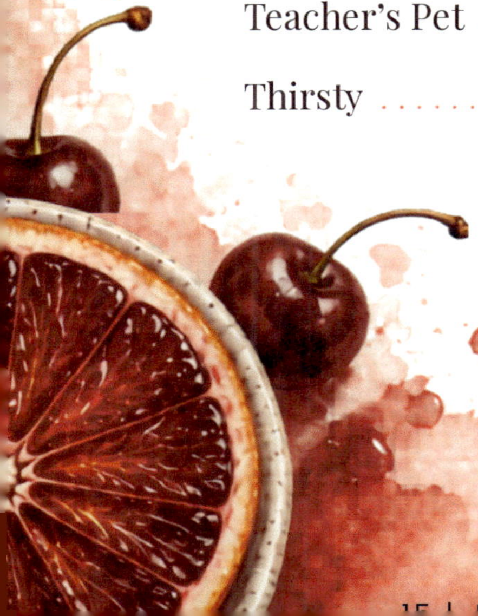

RED MOODS

Bloody Nose

When you want to
give your taste buds
a healthy punch.

The Low Down

This juice has attitude. Bloody Nose is for the days when you're not tiptoeing into the morning. You're charging in. It's bold, it's loud, and it doesn't care if you're ready.

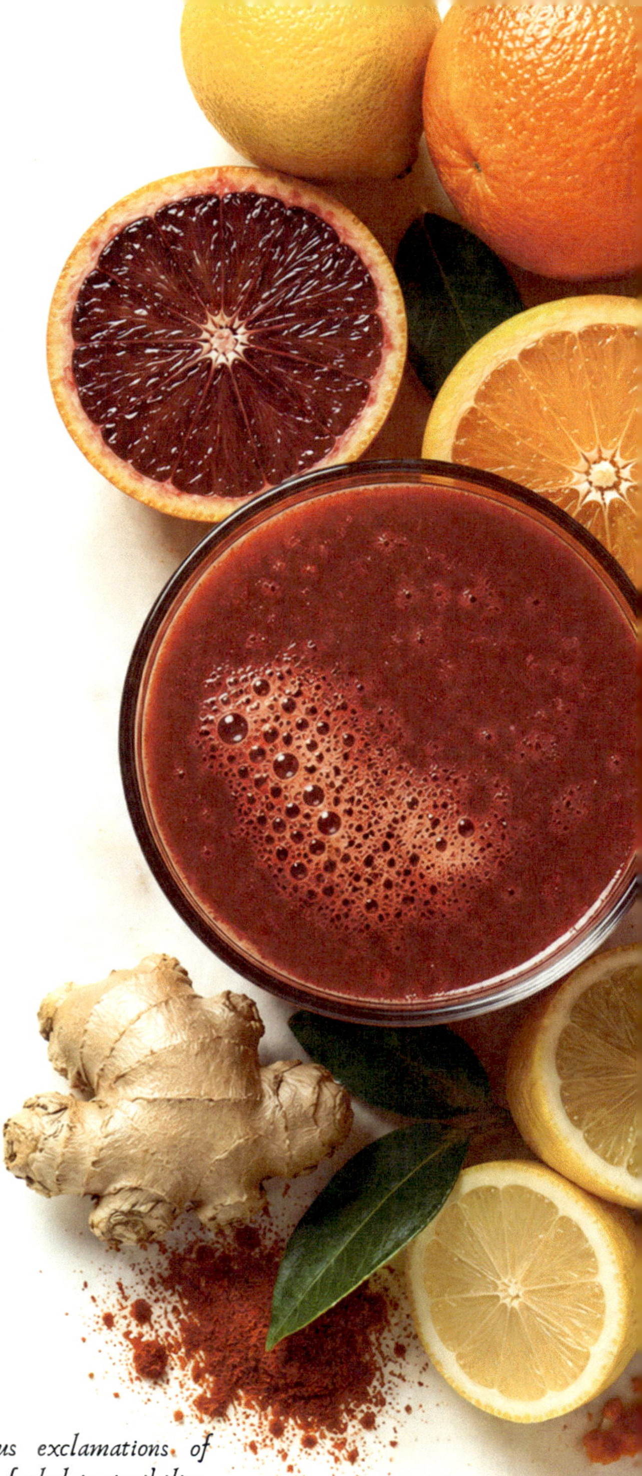

Flavor Profile

A punchy mix of bold orange, sharp lemon, and warm ginger for a lively citrus hit.

Ingredients

- 3 blood oranges, peeled
- 2 large navel oranges, peeled
- 1 lemon, peeled
- 1 inch piece of ginger
- or cayenne pepper (optional)

Perfect For...

Morning energy boosts, pre-workout fire, or when regular orange juice just isn't cutting it anymore.

Side effects may include spontaneous exclamations of 'Woohoo!', temporary feelings of citrus-fueled invincibility, and an urge to challenge lemons to a duel. Despite the name, it will not give you or anyone else a bloody nose, but may make you feel like you can take on anything.

RED MOODS

Brave Soul

When you need
liguid courage and
a zesty kick.

The Low Down

Brave Soul is a dare in a glass. Zesty lemon, cool cucumber, and bold cherries. It is for days when you need to channel your inner superhero.

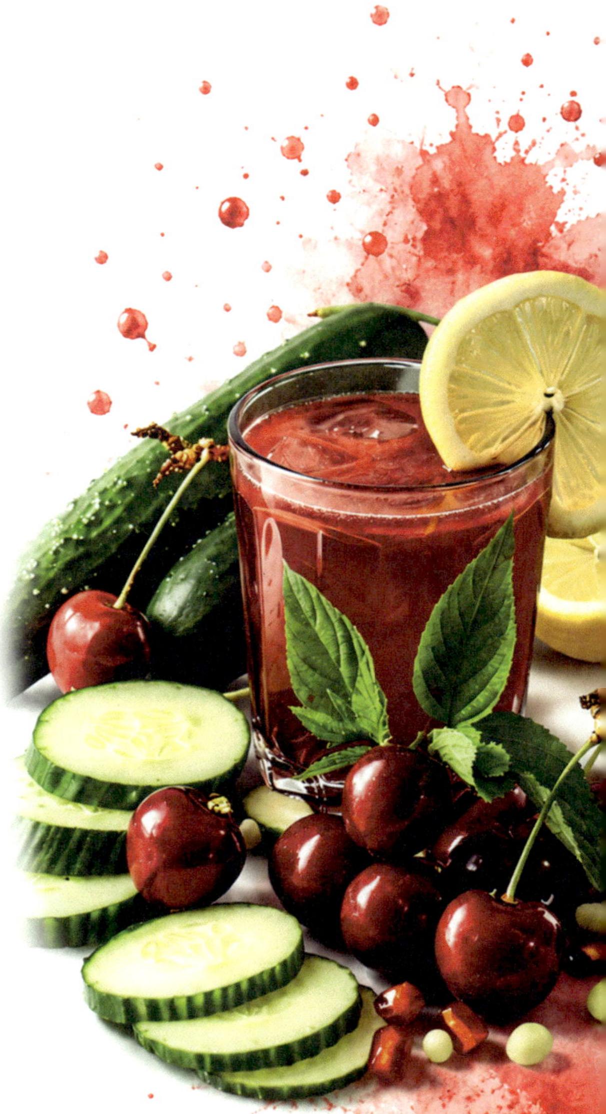

Flavor Profile

Tart, sweet, and refreshing. Like a lemon doing a tango with a cherry while the cucumber plays referee.

Ingredients

- 2 lemons
- 2 cucumbers, peeled
- 1 cup cherries
- 1 tsp cayenne pepper (optional)

Perfect For...

Mornings when you need liquid courage (without the alcohol). Big presentations, first dates, or conquering your to-do list.

Side effects may include sudden urges to skydive, an inexplicable desire to tell your boss what you really think, and the ability to make eye contact with your crush. Consume at your own risk of becoming too awesome.

Chilling Cherry

When you need to
cool down and
sweeten up.

The Low Down

Chilling Cherry is a cozy hug in a glass. Sweet cherries, mellow pear, and a whisper of cinnamon. For days when comfort is the only plan.

Flavor Profile

Deep, sweet cherry flavor with layers of complexity. Bright red cherries, rich black cherries, mellow pear, and a whisper of cinnamon at the edges. Cozy in a glass.

Ingredients

- 2 cups red cherries, pitted
- 2 cups black cherries, pitted
- ½–1 teaspoon cinnamon (stir well)
- 2 pears
- 1 lime, peeled (optional)

Perfect For...

Winding down after a long day, satisfying sweet cravings without the guilt, cozy evenings, or anytime you want a drink that feels like a hug.

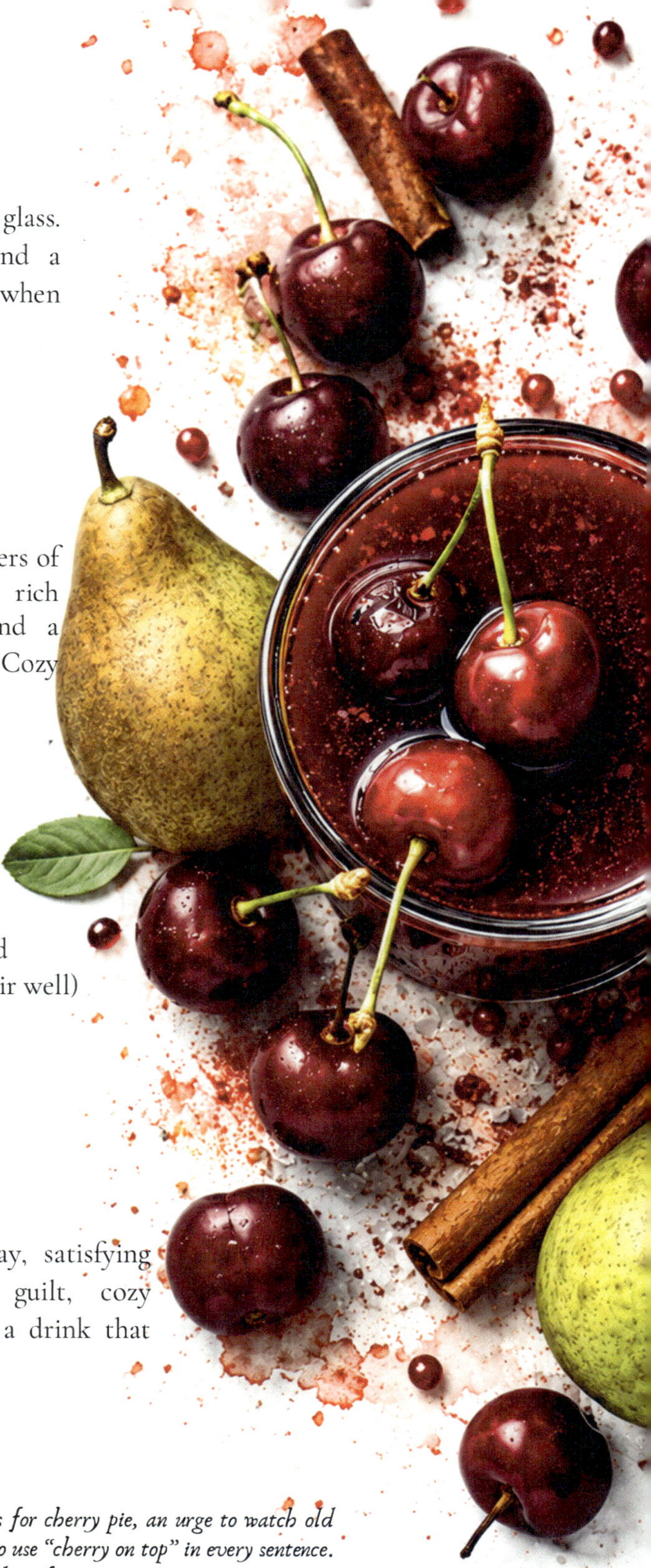

Side effects may include sudden cravings for cherry pie, an urge to watch old movies under a blanket, and the ability to use "cherry on top" in every sentence. May cause unexplained feelings of nostalgia for summers you're not sure you actually had.

RED MOODS

Leaky

When you need a pep talk and your bladder could use some TLC.

The Low Down

Listen up, pee-ple! Leaky is here to make your bathroom visits a VIP experience. This cranberry-based blend is like a spa day for your urinary tract. Refreshing, rejuvenating, and ready to shake out the competition.

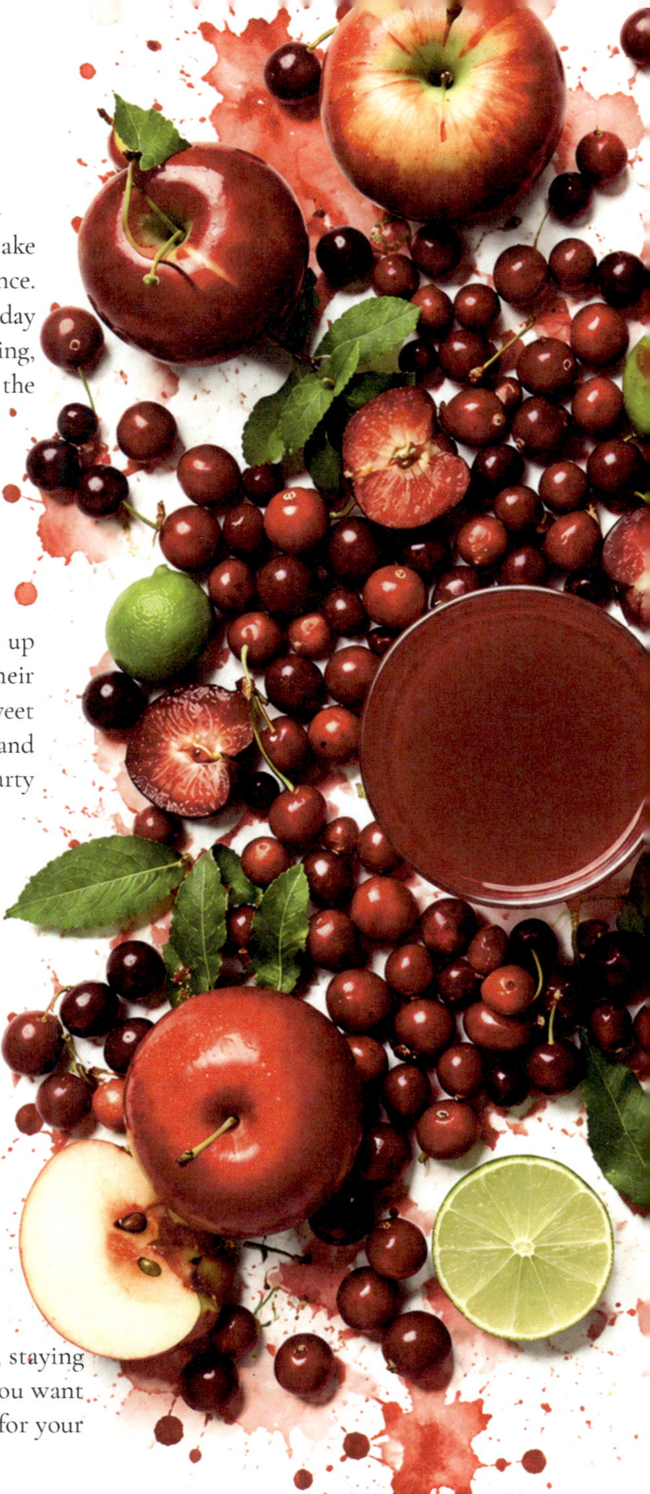

Flavor Profile

A tart and tangy symphony that wakes up your taste buds. Cranberries lead with their signature zing, red apples bring sweet balance, cherries add fruity richness, and lime adds a citrusy kick. It's a fruit party where your kidneys are the VIP guests.

Ingredients

- 1 cup cranberries
- 2 red apples
- 1 cup cherries
- 1 lime, peeled

Perfect For...

Showing your urinary system some love, staying hydrated, and pre-gaming for anytime you want to feel like you're doing something nice for your insides.

Side effects may include frequent trips to the tanning salon, an inexplicable urge to give your restroom a pep talk, and a tendency to overshare about your habits. Not an excuse to avoid drinking water.

RED MOODS

Red Flag

When your uterus
throws a tantrum
and you need to
wave the red flag

The Low Down

This beet-based blend is like a care package for your insides. It is packed with nutrients to help you weather the storm.

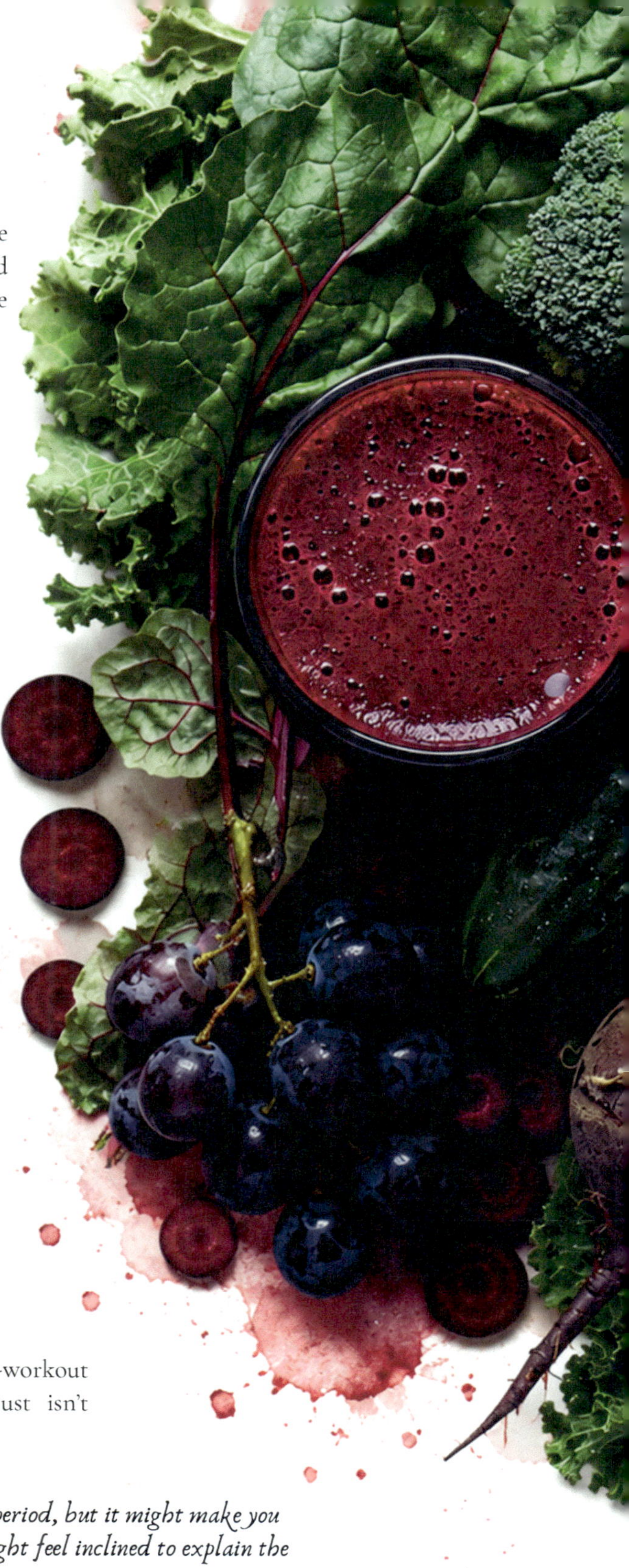

Flavor Profile

A rich, earthy symphony with a hint of sweetness. The beets provide a deep, robust base, while spinach and kale add a green freshness. Cucumber brings a cool, hydrating note, ginger kicks in with a spicy warmth, and dark grapes round it out with a touch of natural sweetness.

Ingredients

- 2 small beets
- 2 cups spinach
- 2 cups kale
- 1 cucumber, peeled
- 2 cups dark grapes
- ¼ inch ginger (optional)
- 1 orange, peeled (optional)

Perfect For...

Morning energy boosts, red days, pre-workout fire, or when regular orange juice just isn't cutting it anymore.

This drink will not actually stop your period, but it might make you feel like you can conquer it, and you might feel inclined to explain the benefits of beets.

RED MOODS

Teacher's Pet

When you're ready to
ace the day.

The Low Down

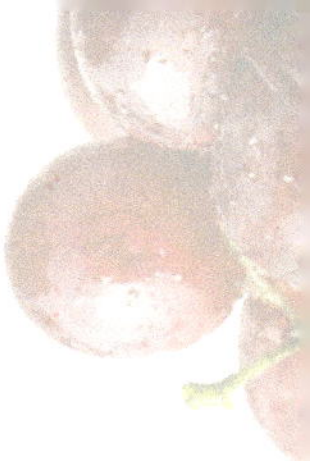

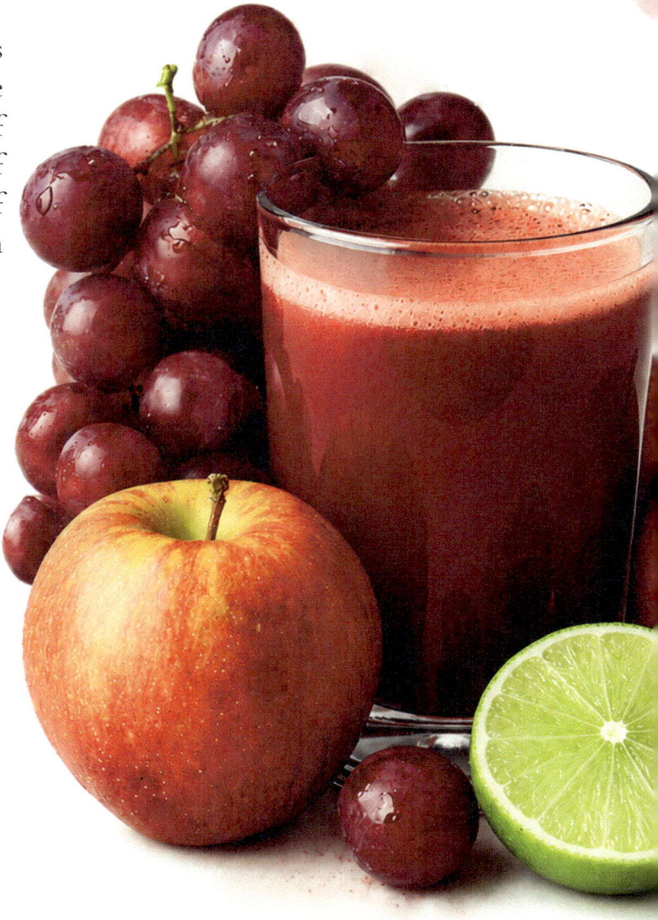

Forget just polishing apples. This is the ultimate way to score brownie points! Teacher's Pet is the A+ of juices, the valedictorian of refreshment, the overachiever of taste. It's so good, it might just earn you extra credit in the game of life!

Flavor Profile

Imagine if an apple and a grape decided to collaborate on a group project, with lime as their sassy study buddy. It's sweet, tart, refreshing, and it's the flavor equivalent of acing a pop quiz you didn't even know you were taking.

Ingredients

- 4 red apples (medium)
- 2 cup red grapes
- 1 lime, peeled

Perfect For...

Staying sharp, feeling steady, or giving yourself a tiny spark when the day gets busy.

Side effects may include sudden urges to raise your hand, a desire to sit in the front row, and the ability to smile wide in life. Consuming this juice does not guarantee actual teacher's-pet status or improved grades.

RED MOODS

Thirsty

When you're parched
and need it to be
obvious.

The Low Down

Sometimes you don't need fancy. You just need water. Melon water. Thirsty is hydration in its purest, most delicious form. It's the drink equivalent of jumping into a pool on a hot day.

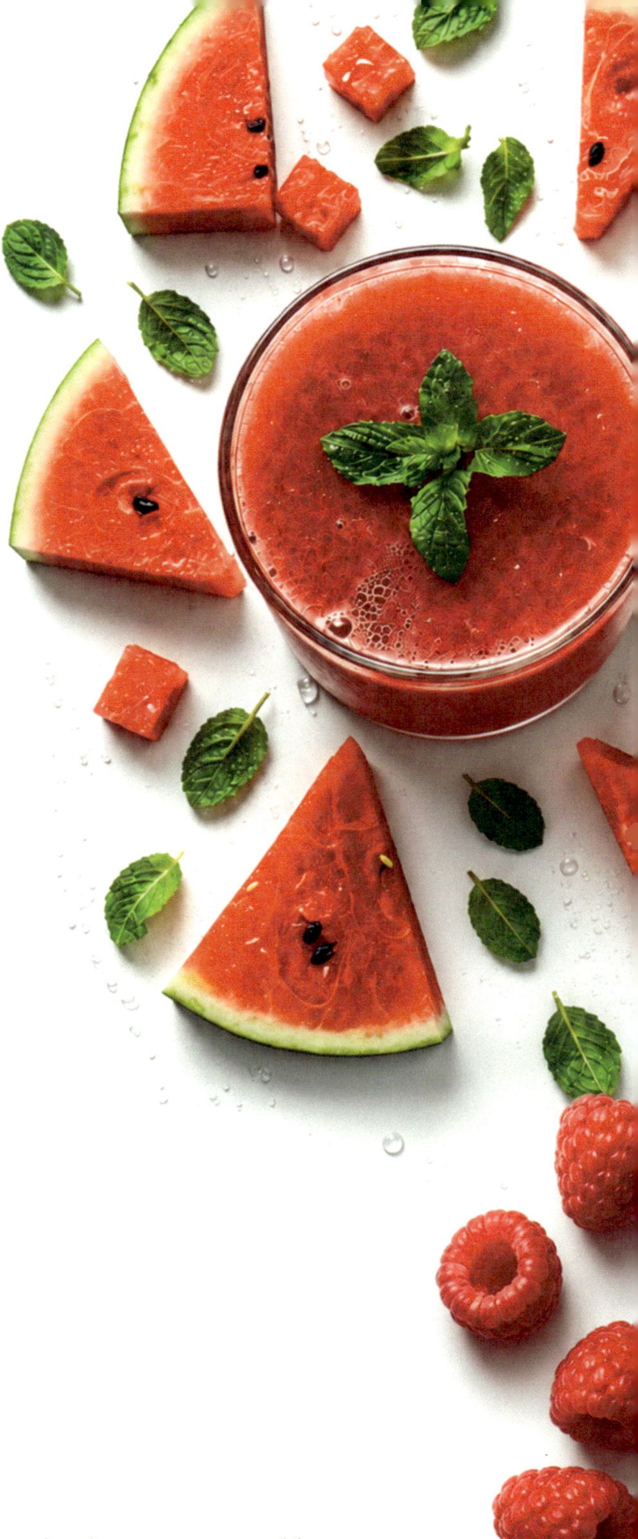

Flavor Profile

Sweet, light, and incredibly refreshing. Mint adds a cool whisper, lime brings zing, but watermelon is the star, and it knows it.

Ingredients

- 4 cups watermelon
- ½ lime, peeled (optional)
- 5-6 mint leaves or a small sprig of mint
- ½ cup raspberries

Perfect For...

Hot days, post-workout cooldowns, when you're thirsty, or anytime you want something sweet without any of the guilt.

Side effects may include drinking the entire batch in one sitting, sudden urges to buy a bigger watermelon, and the realization that you've been overcomplicating hydration your whole life.

You've
fired up.

Now it's time
to go deep.

Purple Moods

Reflective, calming, and brain-friendly

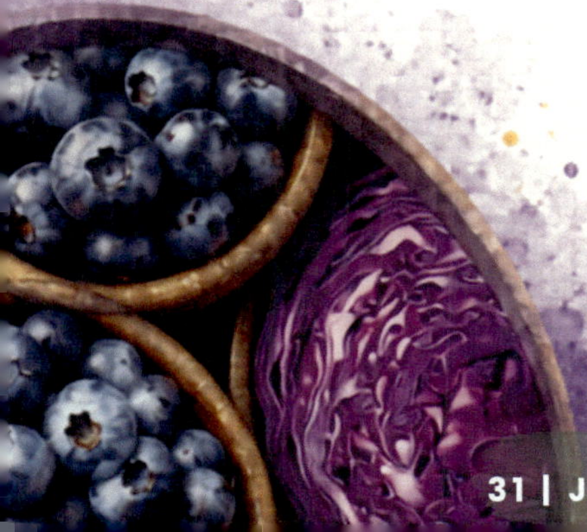

PURPLE MOODS

Beet Down

When you're feeling beat and you need something grounding to bring you back center.

The Low Down

Some days you need to feel your feet on the ground. Beet Down is for the moments when you're scattered, drained, or just tired of floating through the day. It pulls you back to the center. Steady, solid, rooted.

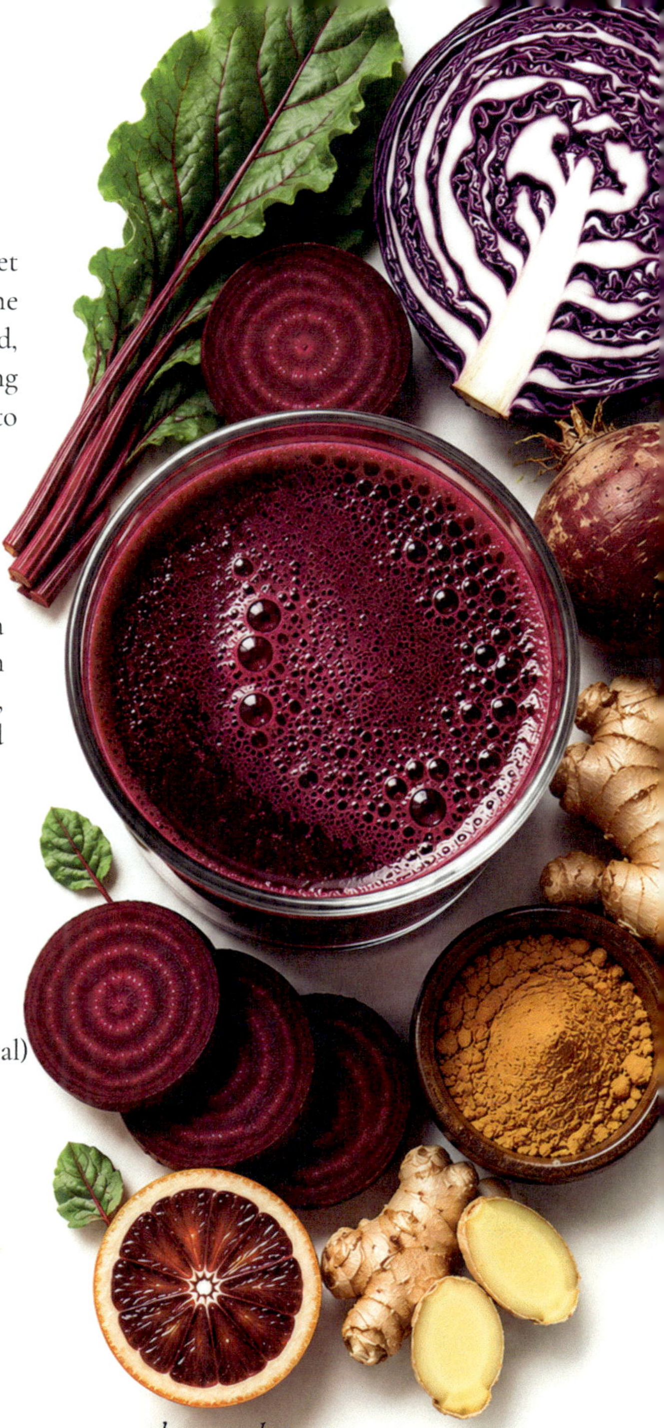

Flavor Profile

Earthy and grounding, with a subtle sweetness from beets, a fresh bite from cabbage, and a warm, gentle finish from ginger and turmeric.

Ingredients

- 4 small beets
- 1 cup chopped red cabbage
- 1-inch piece of ginger
- 1/2 tsp turmeric powder
- 1 blood orange, peeled (optional)

Perfect For...

When you need to fight off the blahs, knock out a case of the Mondays, or want to feel like you're winning at adulting.

Side effects may include a sudden urge to paint everything purple, an inexplicable desire to start a root-vegetable rock band, and the ability to detect vampires from a mile away (garlic, who?). Consumption at your own risk of becoming too healthy.

PURPLE MOODS

Deep

When you need to
slow down and sink
into your feelings.

The Low Down

Sometimes you need to feel your feelings, and Deep is here to sit with you in the blue. This deep, moody blend is smooth, soulful, and a little chill in the best way. It's permission to slow down and process.

Flavor Profile

Rich and velvety with deep berry sweetness. Grapes bring nostalgic childhood-grape-juice depth, purple cabbage adds an earthy depth you can't quite place. Ginger whispers warmth at the end, like a friend resting a hand on your shoulder.

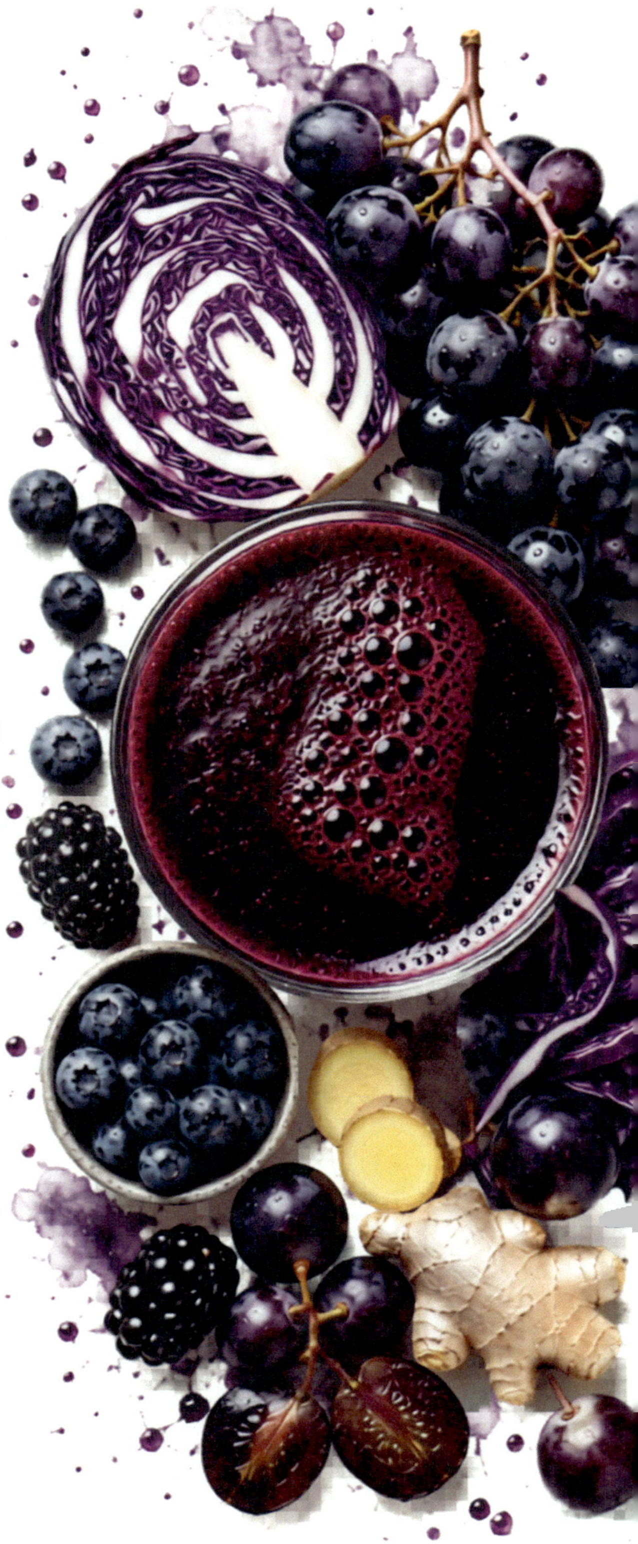

Ingredients

- 1 cup blueberries
- 1 cup blackberries
- 2 cups concord (dark) grapes
- 1 cup purple cabbage
- 1 inch ginger

Perfect For...

Rainy afternoons, processing a tough week, creative blocks that need gentle nudging, or anytime you need to honor a slower pace.

Side effects may include sudden urges to listen to jazz, staring out rain-streaked windows, and writing poetry you'll never show anyone. May cause temporary contentment with doing absolutely nothing.

PURPLE MOODS

Night Owl

When your best ideas come after midnight.

The Low Down

For the late-night thinkers, the 2 am creators, the ones who do their best work when the world goes quiet. Night Owl is dark, bold, and a little mysterious, just like your browser history at 3 am.

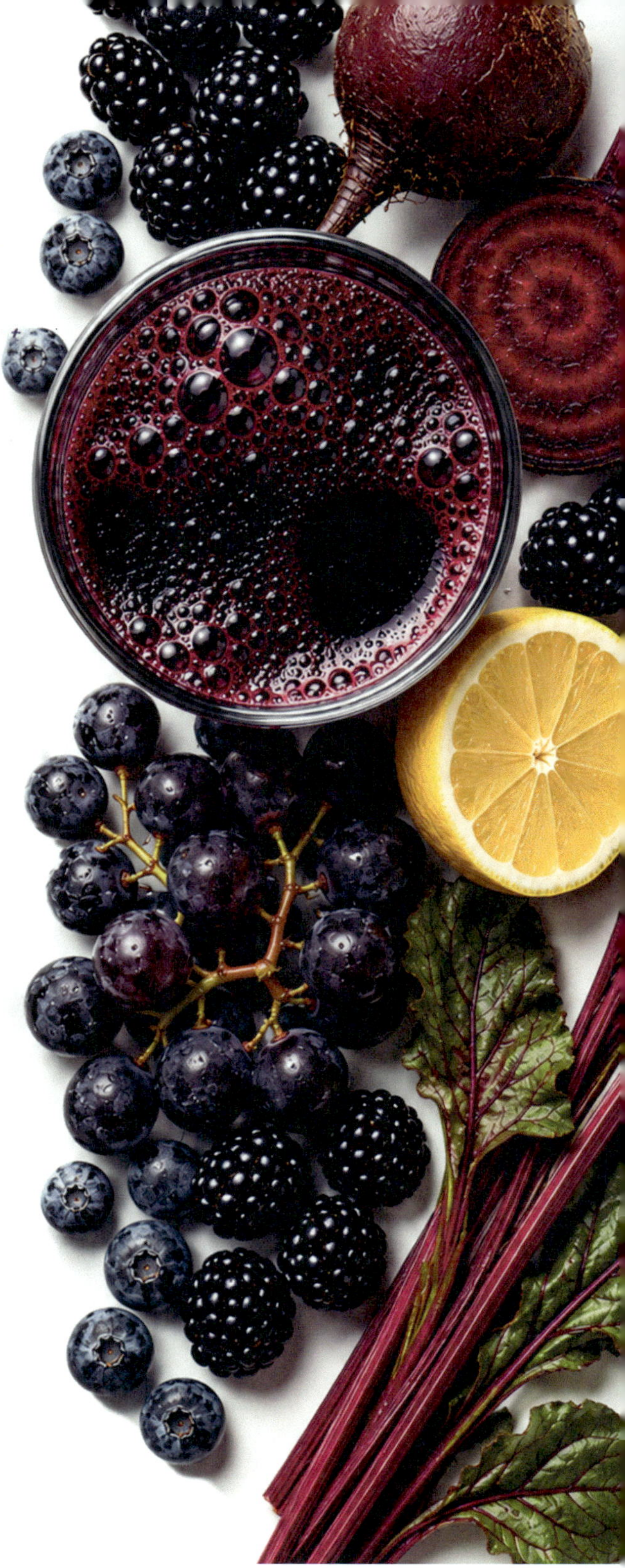

Flavor Profile

A tartness that keeps you alert. The beef adds earthiness and a striking color that looks almost black in the right light. Lemon cuts through with a bright edge, keeping the whole thing from being too brooding. It's serious but not heavy.

Ingredients

- 1/2 cup blackberries
- 1/2 cup blueberries
- 2 cups black grapes
- 1 small beet
- 1 lemon, peeled

Perfect For...

Late-night work sessions, creative breakthroughs, stargazing, deep conversations, or anytime your brain refuses to turn off, and you decide to just go with it.

This isn't a bedtime drink; it's fuel for the minds that come alive after dark. Side effects may include spontaneously solving problems you weren't even working on, and a sudden conviction that you should learn to play the piano.

PURPLE MOODS

Purple Reign

When you are ready
to own the room

The Low Down

Bow to the king of berry juices. Purple Reign is for days when you need to walk in like you own the place, even if "the place" is just your kitchen. It's regal, antioxidant-rich, and has main-character energy. Crown not included, but heavily implied.

Flavor Profile

Bold, tangy, and luxurious. The black grapes bring deep, wine-like richness, pomegranate adds jewel-toned tartness, blueberries round it out with sweetness, and lime keeps things from getting too precious. It tastes expensive. It tastes important.

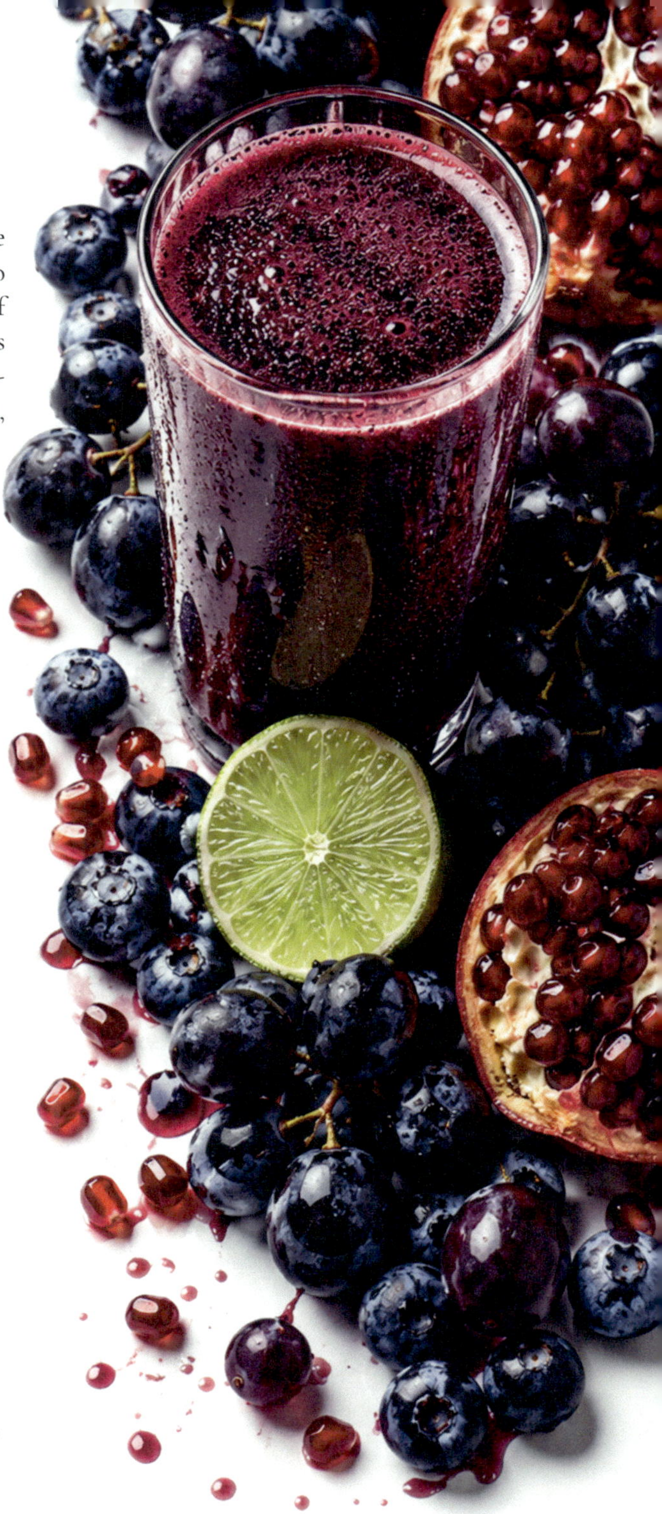

Ingredients

- 2 cups black grapes
- 1 cup blueberries
- 1/2 cup pomegranate seeds
- 1/2 lime, peeled

Perfect For...

When you need to remind yourself you're that person, or anytime you want to feel like royalty without the responsibility of running a kingdom.

Side effects may include walking in slow motion, referring to yourself in the third person, and an inexplicable urge to make a grand entrance everywhere you go. May cause overconfidence in karaoke abilities.

PURPLE MOODS

Smarty Pants

When you need a
mental boost and
want to feel smugly
healthy.

The Low Down

Welcome to the berry-picked path to relaxation! 'Smarty Pants' isn't just a drink; it's nature's chill pill in liquid form. Capture the essence of tranquility and bottle it up with a whole bunch of berries on top!

Flavor Profile

Bright berry sweetness with a smooth, mellow finish. You won't taste the broccoli, just a juicy, fruit-forward thick blend that feels like a treat.

Ingredients

- 1 cup Strawberries
- 1 cup Raspberries
- 1 cup Blue Berries
- 2 1/2 cups Black Grapes
- 1 Pear
- 2 red apples
- 1/2 cup Broccoli

Perfect For...

Evening wind-down, stress relief, or anytime you need to hit the pause button on life's chaos while simultaneously giving your brain a boost. It's the drink equivalent of a yoga session for your neurons!

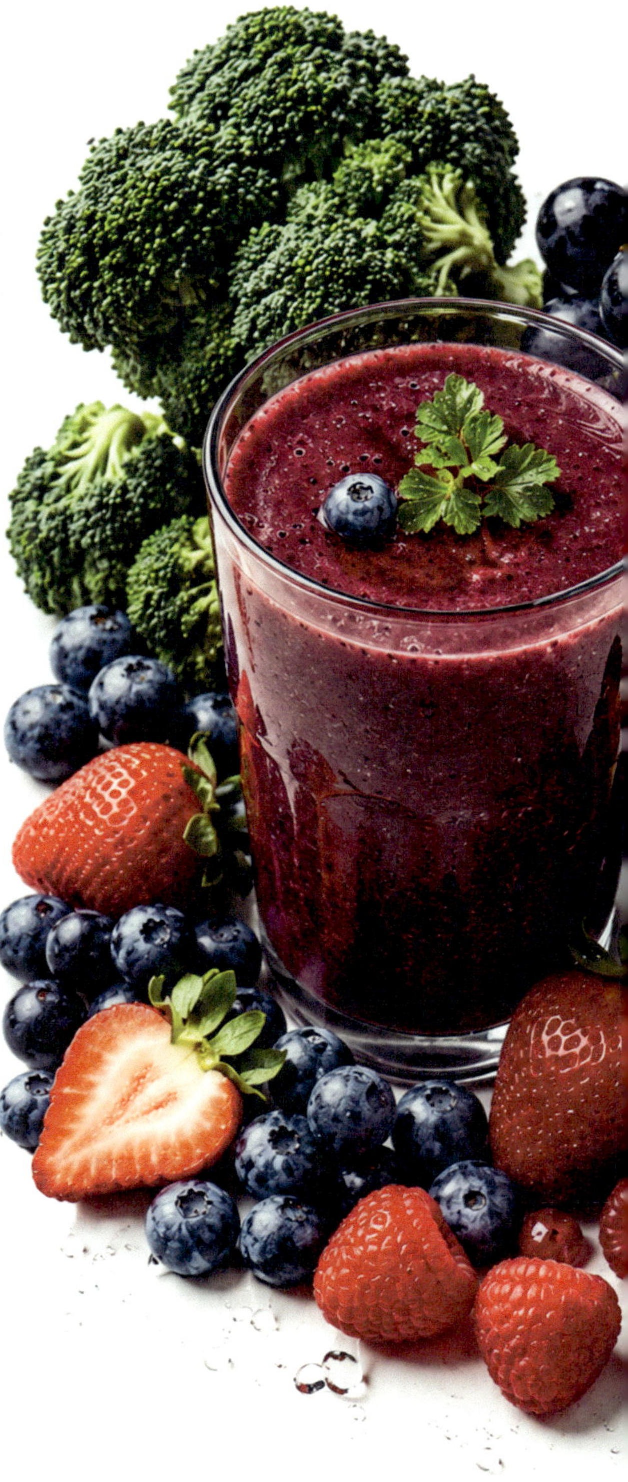

Side effects may include sudden urges to solve complex equations, a strong urge to learn a new language, or the ability to finally understand what your cat is thinking.

PURPLE MOODS

Winey

When you want
wine vibes without
the hangover.

The Low Down

Winey is for grape lovers who want the sophistication of wine without the regret. This all-grape blend is rich, deep, and complex enough to swirl in your glass while pretending you're at a vineyard. Pinky up, health nut!

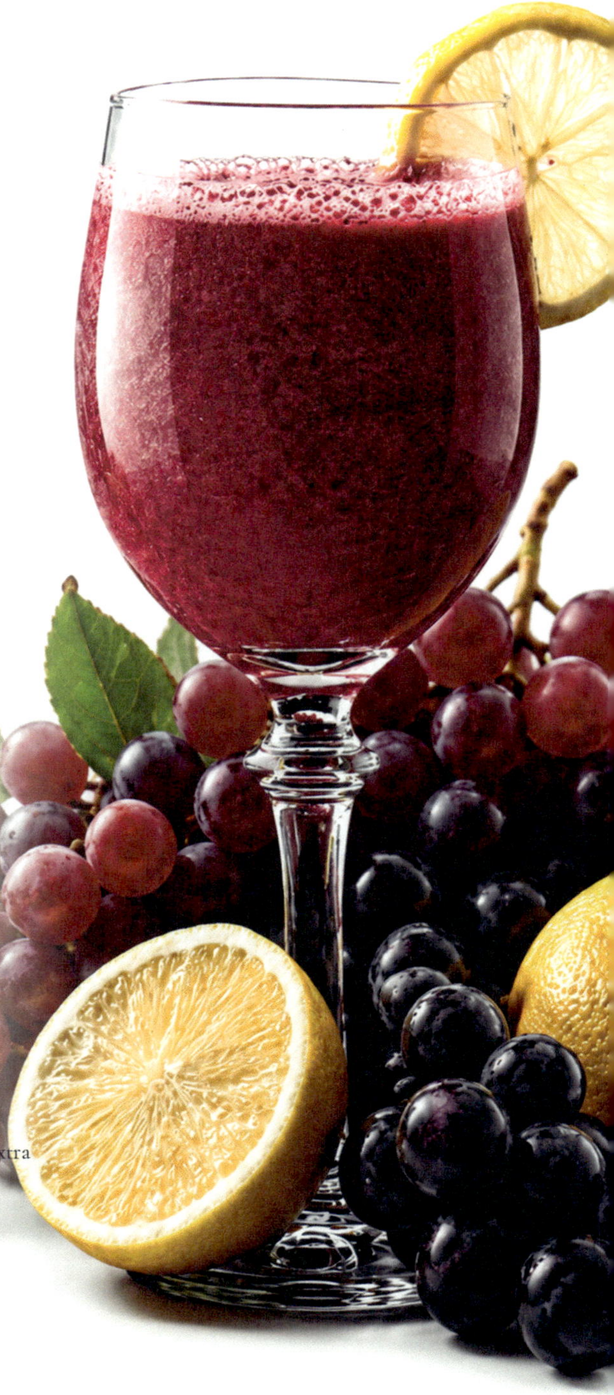

Flavor Profile

Lush and full-bodied with layers of grape sweetness. Red grapes bring bright fruitiness, black grapes add depth and richness, and Concord grapes deliver that nostalgic, almost jammy note, while lemon adds just enough tartness to keep it feeling grown-up.

Ingredients

- 2 cups red grapes
- 1 1/2 cup concord grapes (or black seedless grapes)
- 1 lemon.
- 1 cucumber, peeled

Add a plum and/or a splash of balsamic vinegar for extra wine-like depth.

Perfect For...

Wine lovers doing a cleanse, fancy brunches without the booze, pretending you're more sophisticated than you are, or anytime you want to feel elegant while drinking fruit.

Side effects may include swirling your juice glass, describing flavors with words like "notes" and "undertones," and a sudden urge to visit Napa. Does not actually contain alcohol, but may cause you to act like it does.

Your mood isn't a problem to *fix*. It's just asking for a *drink*.

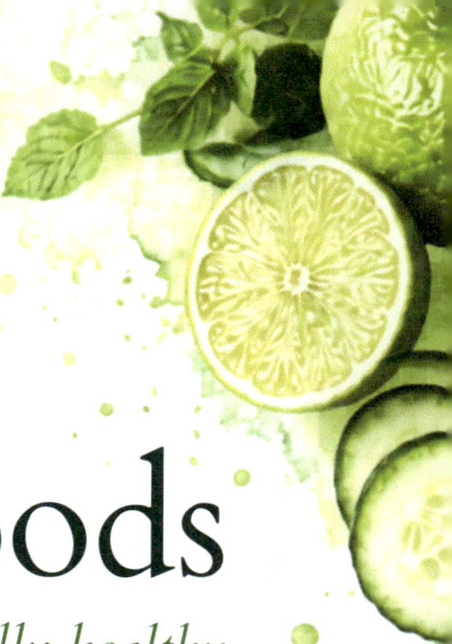

Green Moods

Fresh, leafy, and unapologetically healthy

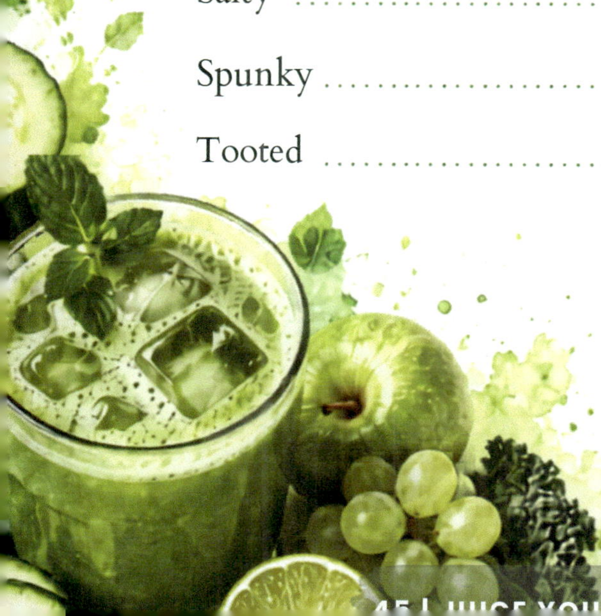

GREEN MOODS

Bitter Grand

When you need a
sophisticated sip
with a little
attitude.

The Low Down

Welcome to the tart side! Bitter Grand isn't just a drink, it's an attitude in a glass. This lip-puckering potion takes your sour mood and turns it into liquid refreshment. It's like giving your taste buds a wake-up call with a megaphone.

Flavor Profile

Tangy and crisp with a hint of earthiness from the rosemary and a sweet note from the grapes.

Ingredients

- 3 granny smith apples
- 1 lemon (peeled)
- 1 rosemary sprig or pinch of ground rosemary
- 1 cup green grapes
- ½ grapefruit, peeled (optional)

Perfect For...

Those days when you want to embrace your inner grouch while secretly nourishing your body. Who said being bitter can't be delicious?

May cause a sudden appreciation for the finer things in life. Consume with a sense of sophistication.

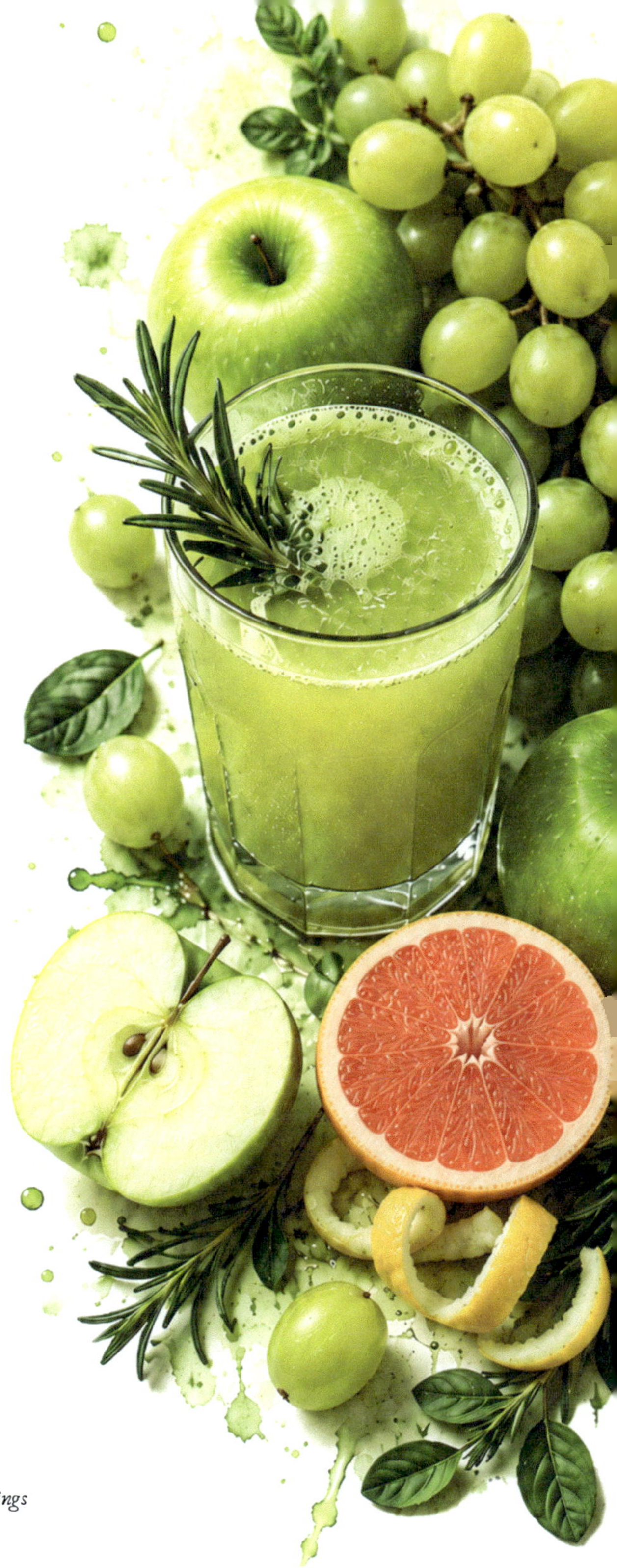

GREEN MOODS

Bloated

When your belly's throwing a tantrum and you need to deflate.

The Low Down

We've all been there, feeling like a balloon animal at a birthday party nobody asked for. Bloated is here to help you release the pressure (with grace). This blend is light, soothing, and ready to calm the chaos happening in your midsection.

Flavor Profile

Cool and refreshing with a tropical brightness. Cucumber and mint keep things calm, pineapple brings natural sweetness, ginger adds gentle warmth, and lemon ties it all together with a citrus lift. It's like a spa day for your gut.

Ingredients

- 2 cucumbers
- 3 cups pineapple chunks
- 1 inch piece of ginger
- 1 lemon, peeled
- A few mint leaves (optional)

Perfect For...

Post-meal puffiness, water-retention days, when your body's holding on to everything, or anytime you need to feel a little lighter.

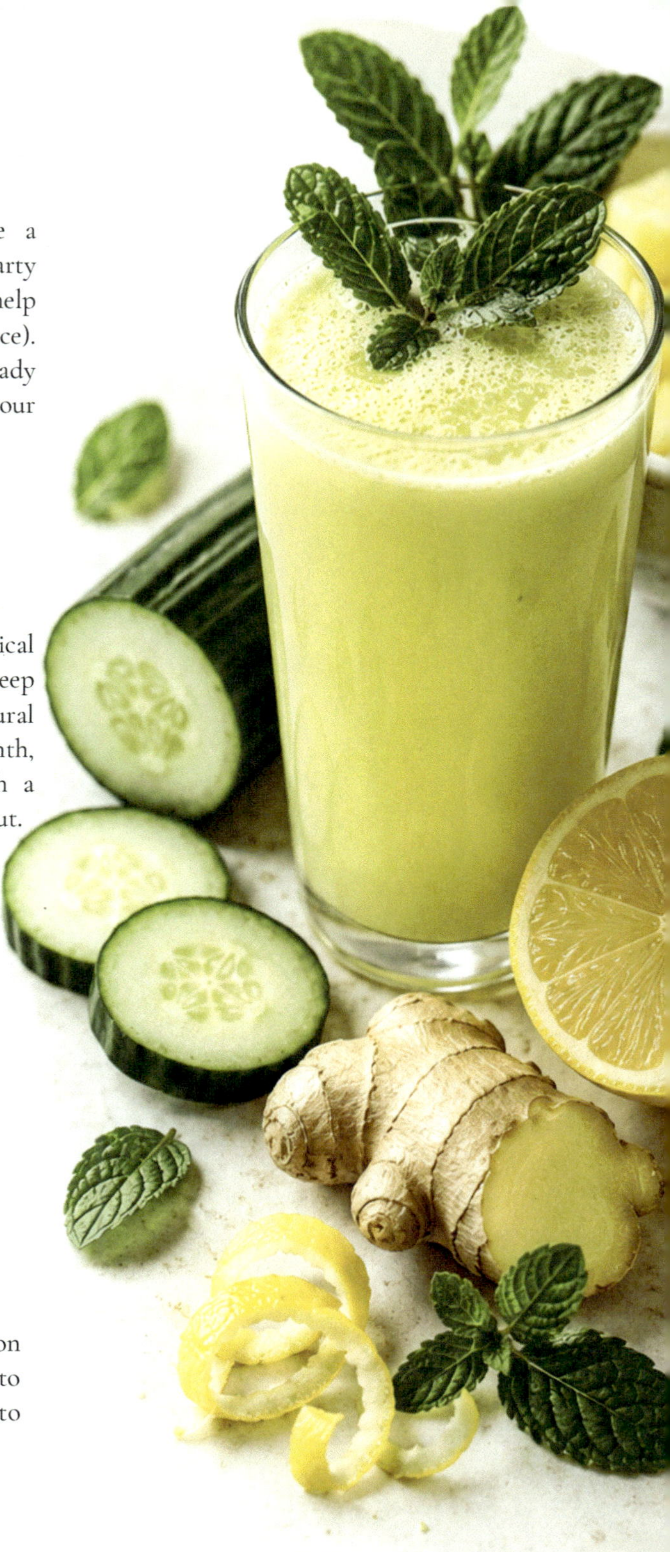

Side effects may include your pants fitting better, an inexplicable urge to unbutton nothing, and the relief of finally feeling like yourself again. May *cause dramatic sighs of comfort.*

GREEN MOODS

Chuckle

When you just
need to lighten up
and have fun.

The Low Down

Psst... this one's all about lighthearted joy. Chuckle brings back that familiar, carefree feeling. Playful, refreshing, and just grown-up enough

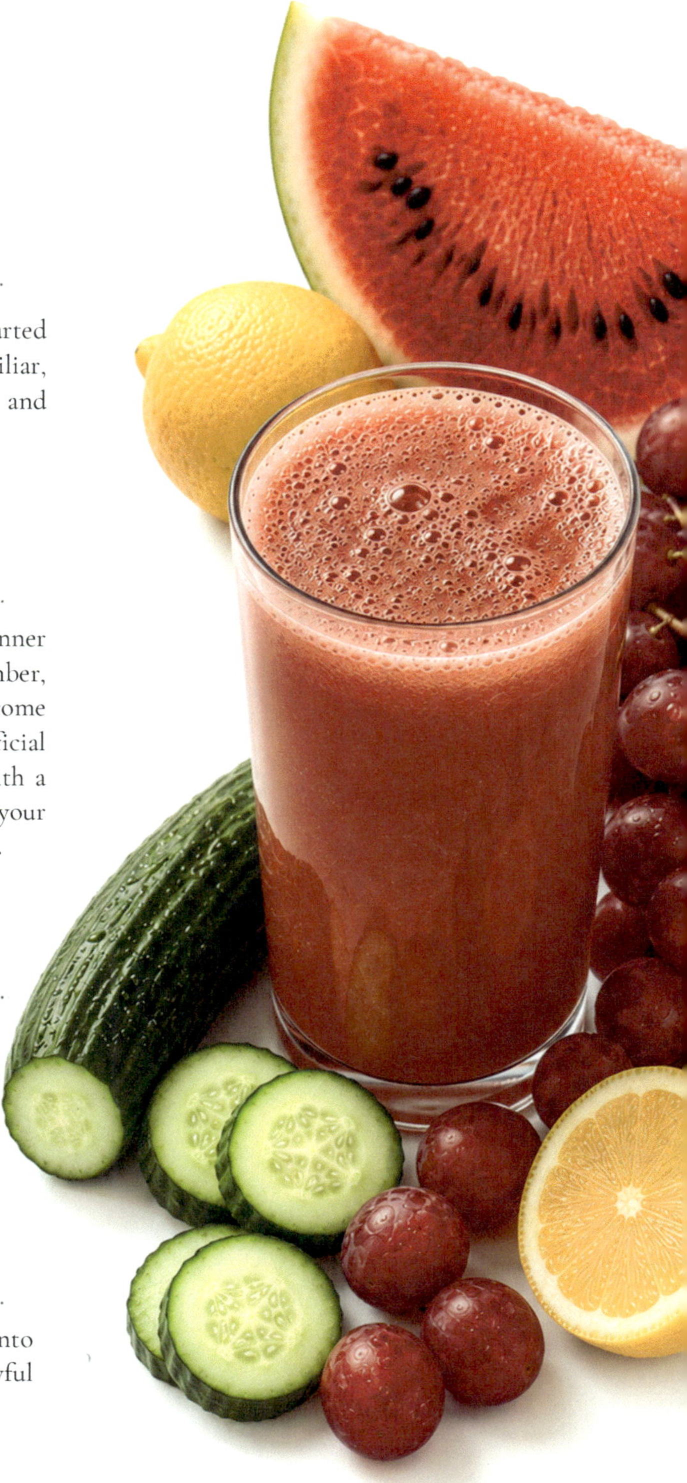

Flavor Profile

A playful blend that wakes up your inner kid. Sweet watermelon, cool cucumber, zippy lemon, and rich red grapes come together in a way that makes artificial flavors seem dull. It's comforting with a clever twist, like discovering your imaginary friend became a comedian.

Ingredients

- 2 cups watermelon
- 2 cucumbers
- 1 lemon, peeled
- 3 cups red grapes

Don't let the color fool you. This one's got green vibes

Perfect For...

Lightening the mood, sneaking into something healthy, and feeling playful without trying too hard

May spark surprise laughter, dad jokes, and unexplained grins. Green drink appreciation may rise. Funny level not guaranteed.

GREEN MOODS

Green Lemonade

When life throws
you lemons,
throw in a
cucumber and
confuse everyone.

The Low Down

Green Lemonade is what happens when a classic decides to grow up, get a spa membership, and still show up refreshing as ever. It's hydration with attitude.

Flavor Profile

A refreshing rollercoaster that starts with the cool, crisp whisper of cucumber, zooms into the zesty zing of lemon, and finishes with the sweet pop of green grapes.

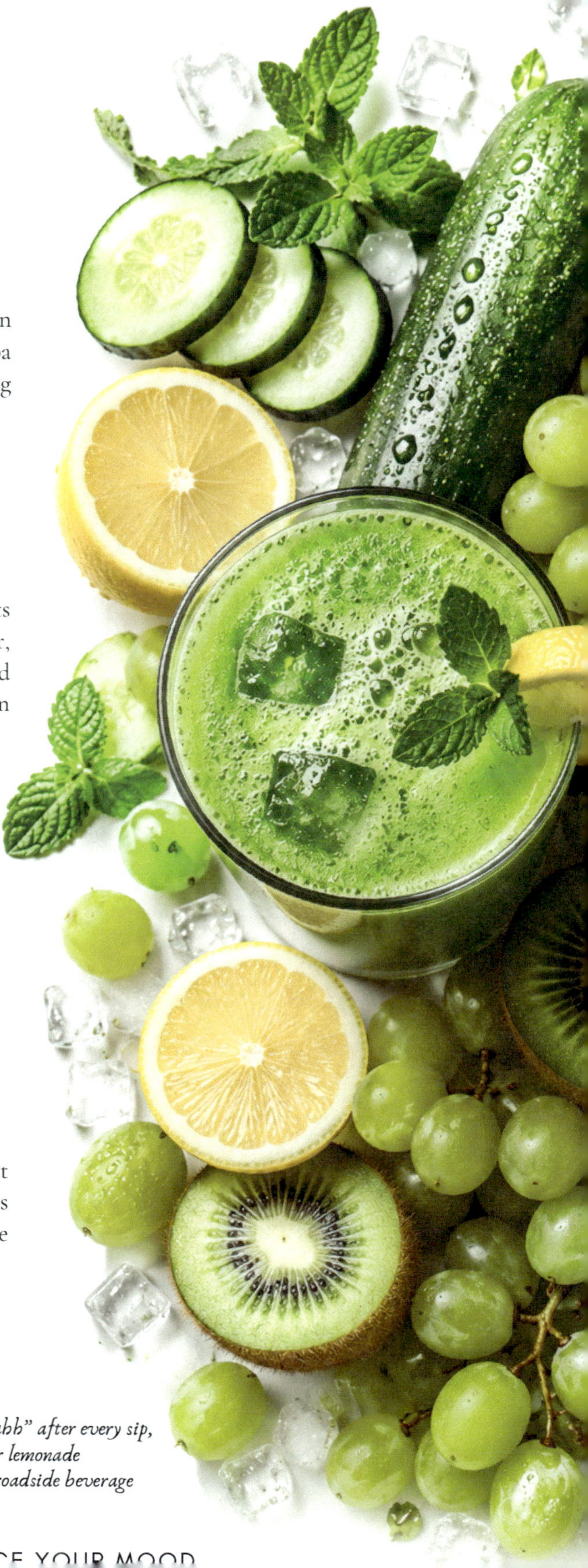

Ingredients

- 2 cucumbers
- 2 lemons or limes, peeled
- 3 cups green grapes
- 3 kiwi fruit

Perfect For...

Hot summer days, post-workout hydration, impressing health-conscious friends, or anytime you want lemonade without the sugar crash.

Side effects may include sudden urges to say "ahh" after every sip, an inexplicable sense of superiority over regular lemonade drinkers, and the confidence to open your own roadside beverage stand.

Green Mustache

When you want
to flex your green
game and wear
your health on
your upper lip.

The Low Down

The Green Mustache is the ultimate green flex. This juice is like a spa day for your cells. This isn't just a juice, it's a leafy green legacy and packed with veggies that say," I care about my health!" A sip of this and you are basically photosynthesizing.

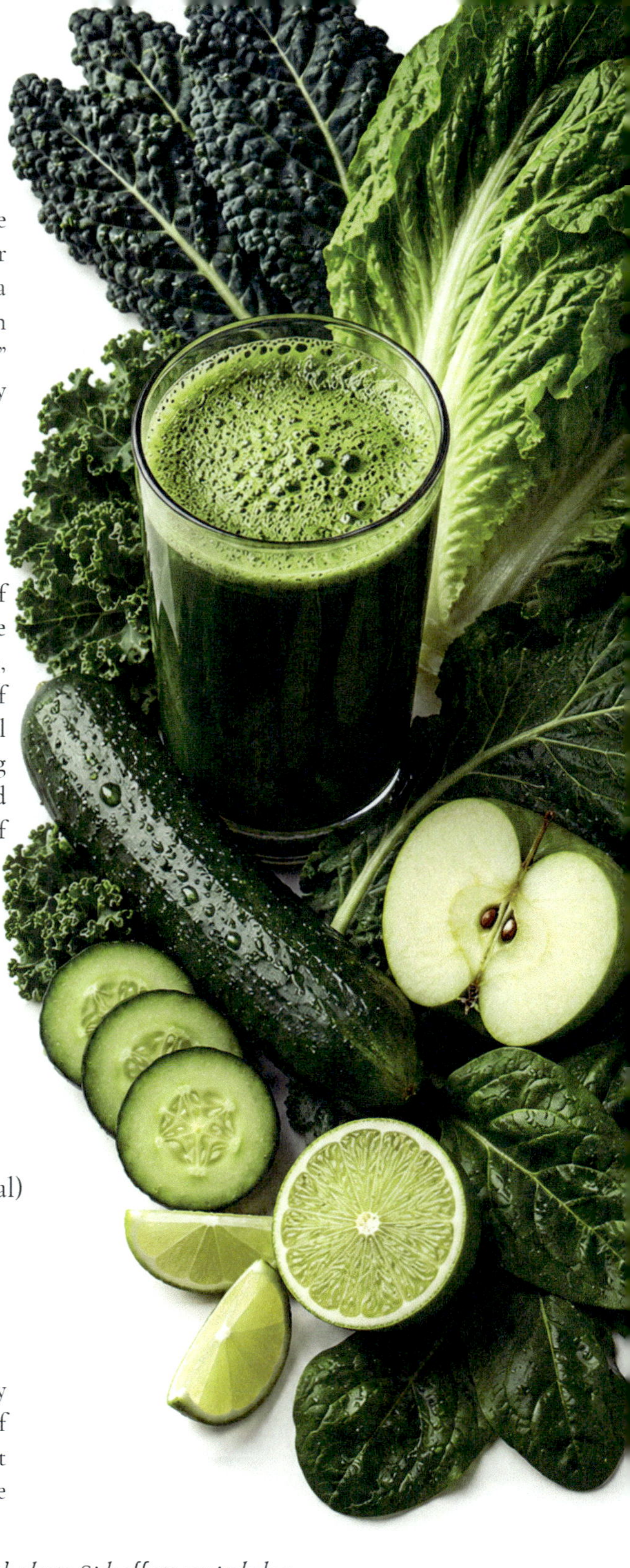

Flavor Profile

It starts with the bold, earthy notes of kale and spinach, swings through the slightly bitter kick of collard greens, mellows out with the crisp freshness of romaine, and finishes with the cool hydration of cucumber. It's like mowing the lawn with your mouth, but in a good way! Each gulp is a green badge of courage for your taste buds.

Ingredients

- 2 cups kale
- 2 cups spinach
- 2 cups chopped collard greens
- 2 cups romaine lettuce
- 2 cucumbers
- 1 lime or lemon, peeled (optional)
- 3 green apples (optional)

Perfect For...

Channeling your inner rabbit (but way cooler). Getting your daily dose of greens without the chewing workout and feeling superior about your veggie intake.

May cause a sudden ability to communicate with plants. Side effects can include a temporary green mustache and an urge to change your name to "Kale or Kaley".

Salty

When you're
feeling salty and
not sorry about it.

The Low Down

Some days you just wake up salty. Instead of fighting it, lean in. This celery-forward juice is crisp, clean, and unapologetically briny. The green apple and grapes add just enough sweetness to take the edge off a little. You're still salty, after all. Everyone else started it.

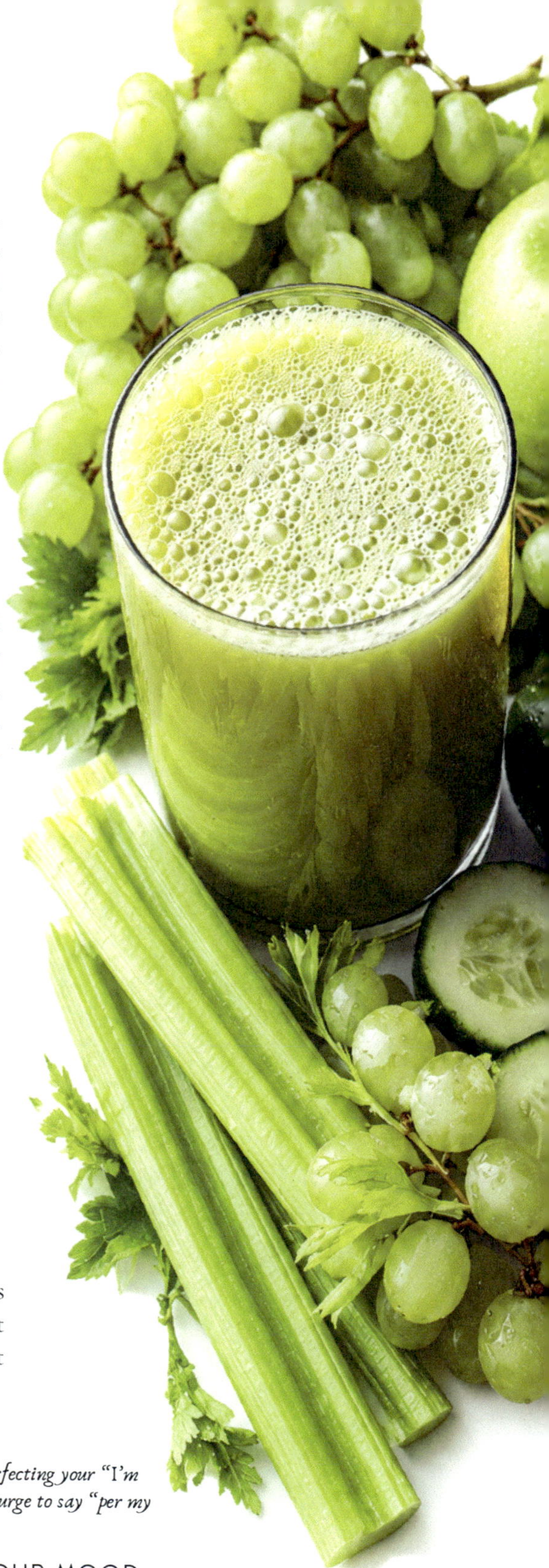

Flavor Profile

Crisp and refreshing with a natural mineral bite from celery, balanced by tart-sweet green apple and juicy grapes. Cucumber adds cool hydration, lemon brightens it up. Clean, simple, no-nonsense.

Ingredients

- 4-5 celery stalks
- 2 green apples
- 1 cup green grapes
- 1 cucumber, peeled
- 1/2 lemon, peeled (optional)

Perfect For...

When you're annoyed and hydrated is the only goal. Or when you want something clean and simple without being overly sweet.

Side effects may include side-eyeing everyone, perfecting your "I'm not mad, just disappointed" face, and a sudden urge to say "per my last email." Pairs well with Monday mornings.

Spunky

When you need a
little kick with no
complications.

The Low Down

Simple. Sharp. No-nonsense. Spunky is for the days when you don't need much, just a little zing to keep you moving.

Flavor Profile

Tart green apple leads with crisp, confident energy. Celery adds cool, mineral backbone. Lemon delivers the snap.

Ingredients

- 4 small green apples
- 2 celery stalks
- ½ lemon, peeled

Perfect For...

When you're low on ingredients but high on attitude, or anytime you want clean, bright energy without overthinking it.

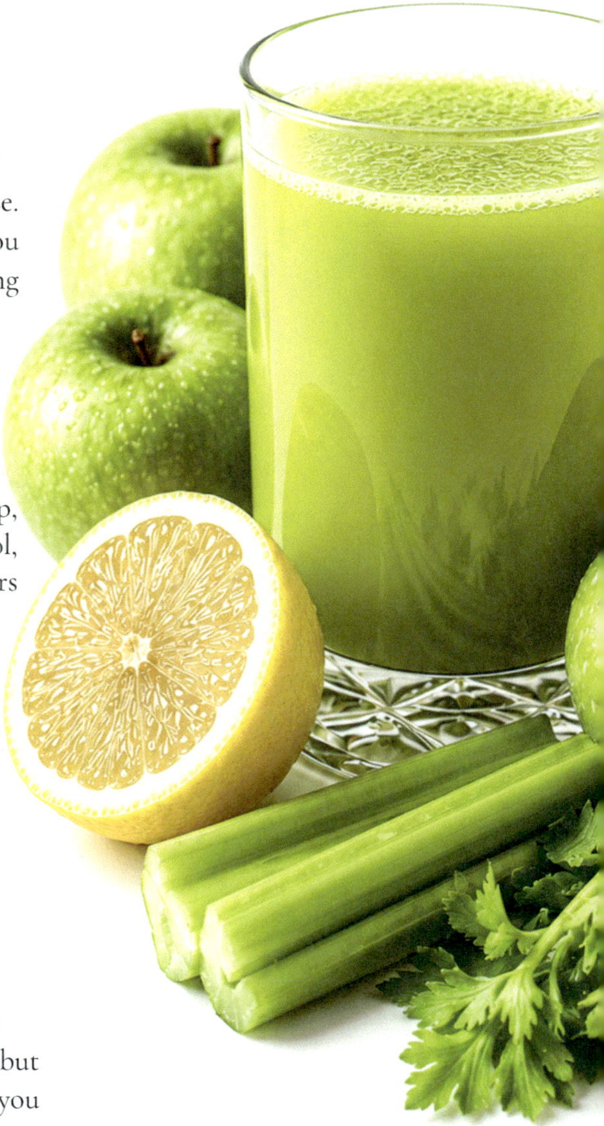

Side effects may include sudden bursts of productivity, saying what you mean, and a suspicious amount of pep in your step.

Tooted

When you need a
detox and don't
mind the
consequences.

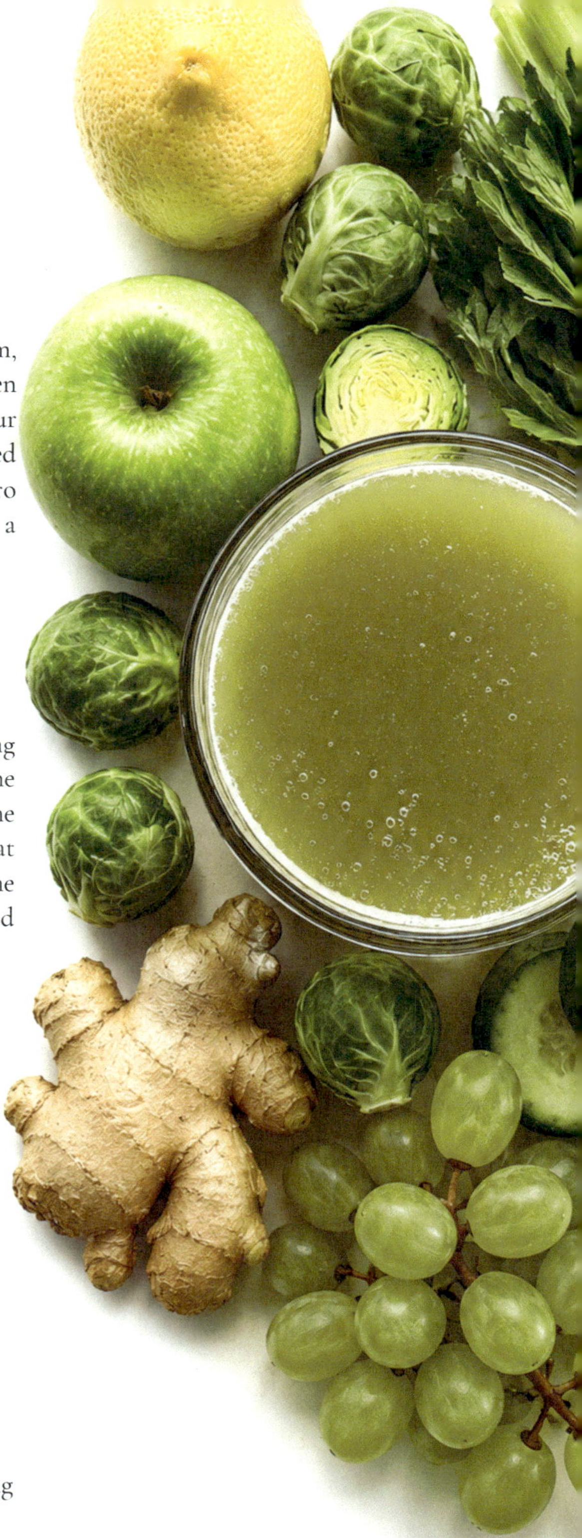

The Low Down

Let's address the elephant in the room, or rather, the toot. Tooted is a green detox powerhouse that will cleanse your system from the inside out. It's packed with fiber and nutrients, with zero apologies. Sometimes getting healthy is a little noisy. Worth it.

Flavor Profile

Green and refreshing with a slight zing from the ginger, balanced by the sweetness of green apple and grapes. The Brussels sprouts add an earthy depth that says "I'm a serious juice," while the cucumber keeps things cool and hydrated

Ingredients

- 2 cups Brussels sprouts
- 2 celery stalks
- 3 green apples
- 1 cucumber
- 2 cups green grapes
- ¼ inch of ginger

Perfect For...

Detox days, reset moments, and letting go of what doesn't serve you.

Consume with a sense of humor and perhaps some alone time. Your gut will thank you; your roommates may not.

A little
energy
can change
everything.

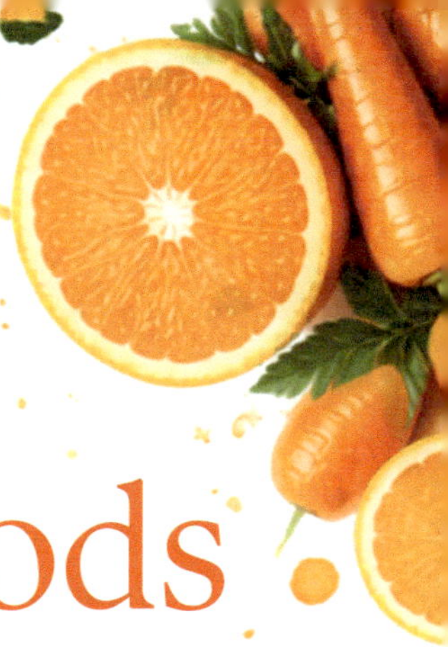

Orange Moods

Zesty, playful, and mood-lifting

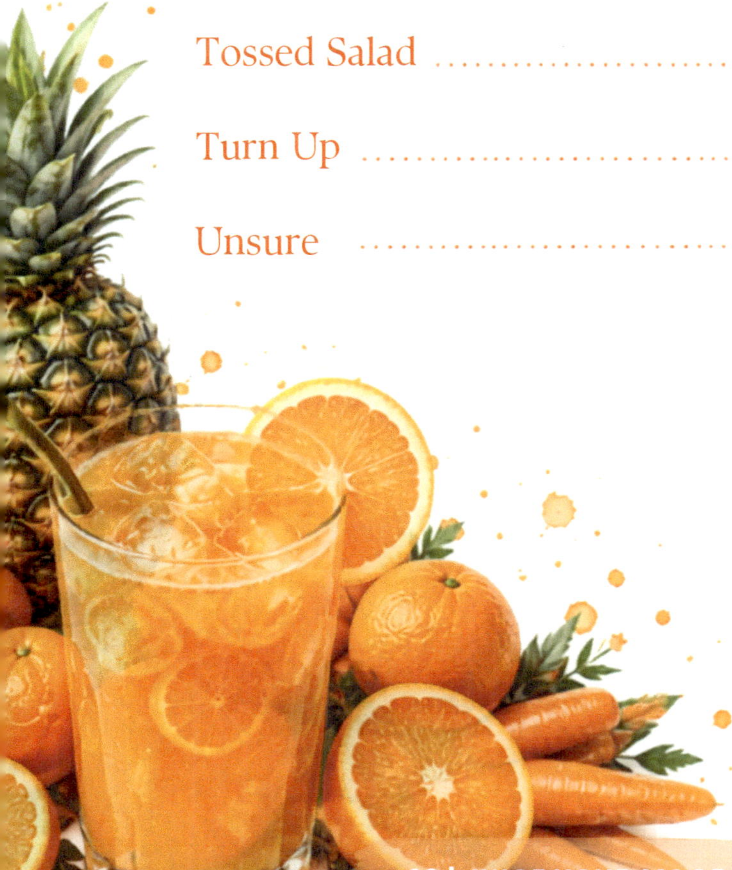

Orange Sucker Punch

When you need a
punch of sunshine
and a roundhouse
of zest.

The Low Down

Orange Sucker Punch isn't your grandma's orange juice (unless your grandma was a secret boxer, in which case, cool grandma!). It delivers a swift, citrusy jab to your taste buds that'll leave you feeling like you've won the flavor championship. It's sunshine in a glass, with an attitude.

Flavor Profile

Bright, bold, and citrusy with a hint of spicy ginger and tropical pineapple. Imagine if an orange decided to take up kickboxing on a beach. It's zesty and invigorating with a punch that'll make your mouth do a double-take.

Ingredients

- 4 large oranges
- 1 cup pineapple
- 1 lemon, peeled
- 1 inch ginger

Perfect For...

A go-to for a morning energy boost, pre-workout hydration, or a refreshing summer cool-down. It satisfies sweet cravings healthily and doubles as a vibrant, non-alcoholic party mixer that's sure to impress.

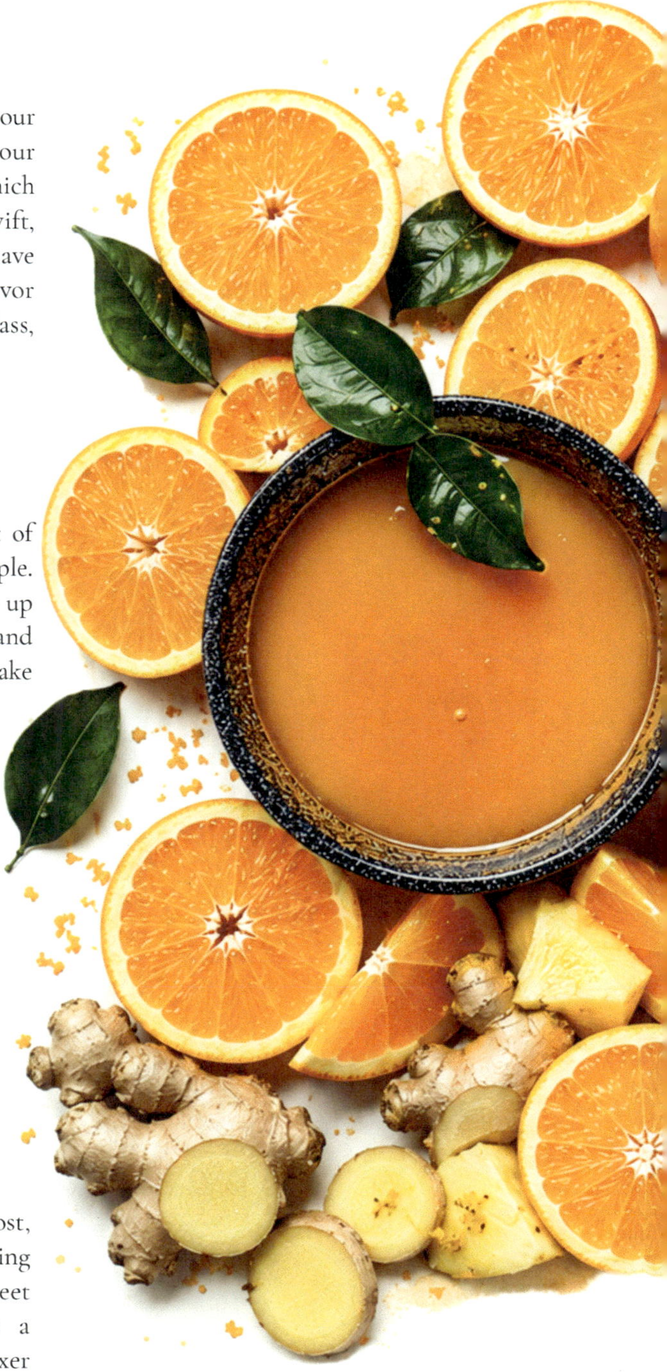

May cause sudden bursts of energy, spontaneous shadow boxing. Consume with caution if you're trying to maintain a grumpy disposition.

ORANGE MOODS

Spicy Carrot

When you want
your vegetables to
bite back.

The Low Down

Spicy Carrot isn't here to play nice. It's the juice that looked at regular carrot juice and said, "That's cute, but watch this."

Flavor Profile

With the sweetness of carrots, the brightness of bell peppers, bright citrus, and tropical pineapple meets a cayenne kick that'll wake up your whole face, this one's for people who like their vegetables with a little attitude.

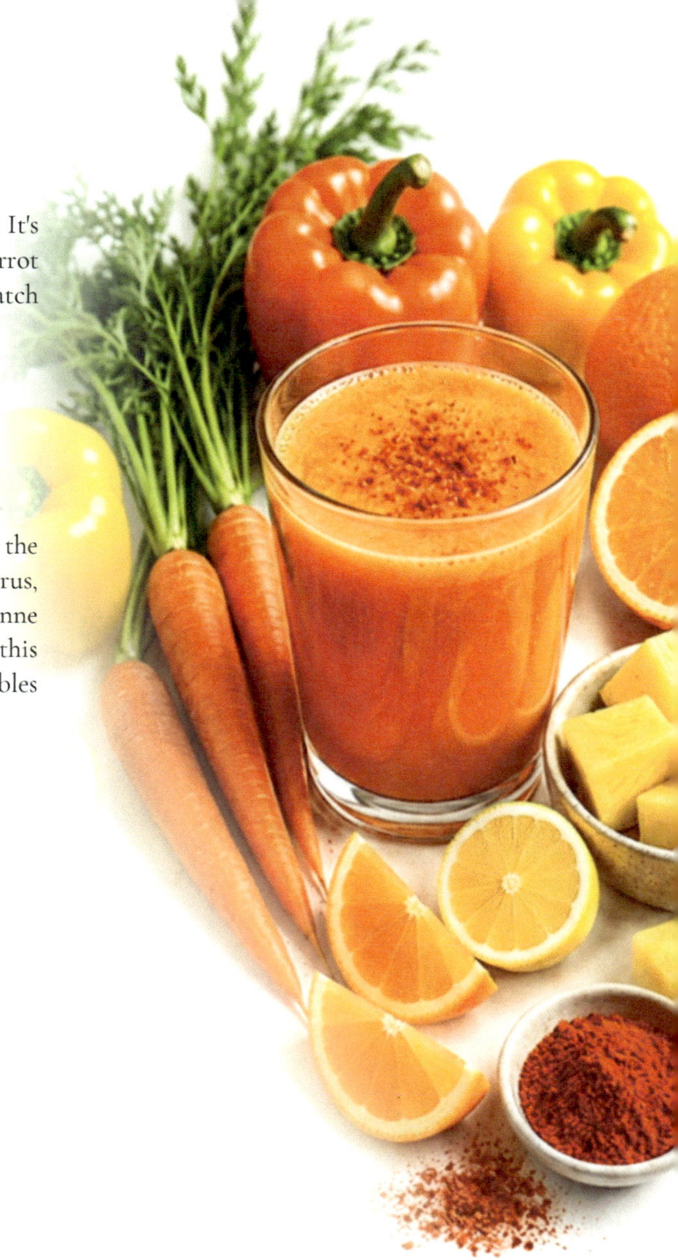

Ingredients

- 4 large carrots
- 1 orange bell pepper
- 1 yellow bell pepper
- 2 oranges
- 1 cup pineapples
- ½ lemon, peeled
- 1 -2 tsps cayenne pepper

Perfect For...

Cold mornings that need a wake-up call, when you're bored with mild flavors, impressing spice-loving friends, or anytime you want your juice to have a personality.

Side effects may include a sudden need to fan your mouth, an urge to add hot sauce to everything, and a newfound respect for carrots as a lifestyle. May cause temporary feelings of invincibility.

ORANGE MOODS

Tossed Salad

When you want to
drink your veggies
and pretend
you're fancy.

The Low Down

Who says you can't drink your salad? Tossed Salad is here to flip the script on your greens routine. It's like your favorite garden party decided to jump into a blender and emerge as the coolest drink in town. No fork required. Just sip your way to veggie victory.

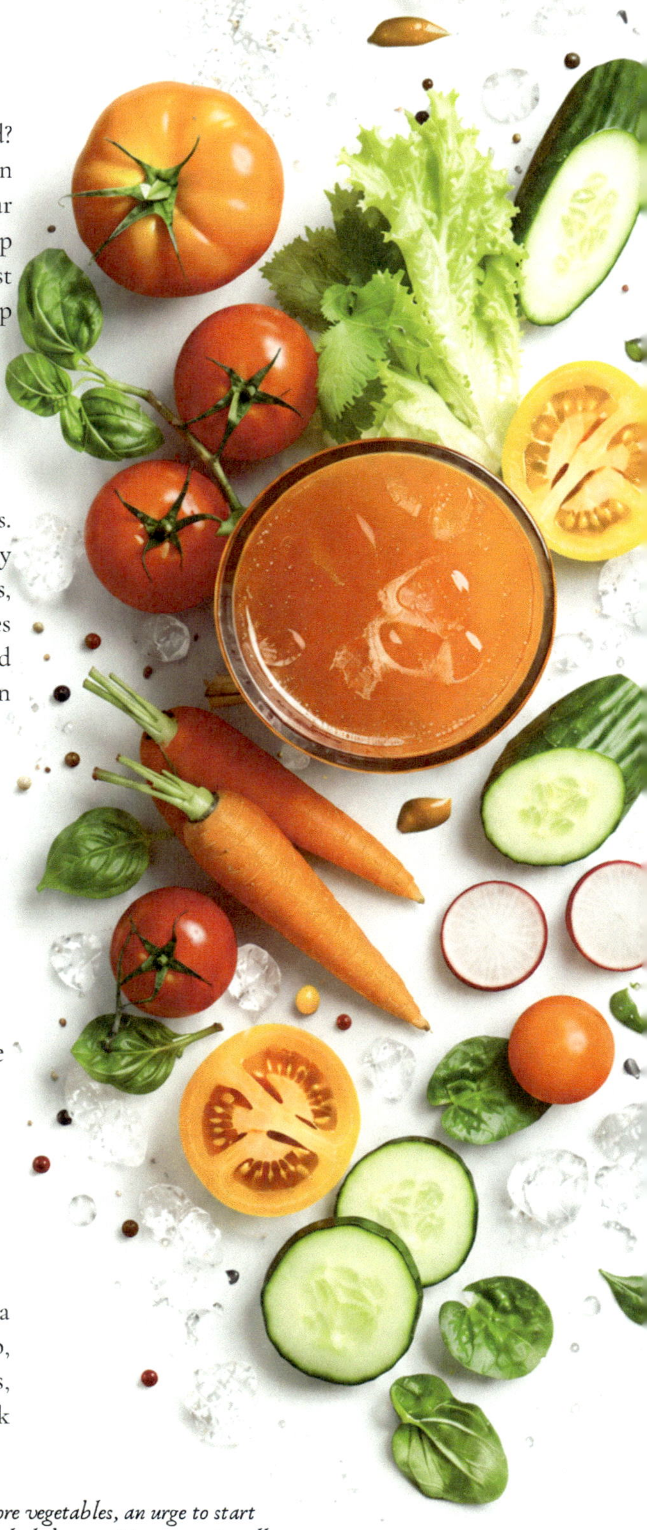

Flavor Profile

A vibrant medley of garden-fresh flavors. Tomatoes provide a sweet and tangy base, cucumbers add a cool crispness, carrots bring subtle sweetness, radishes kick in with a peppery punch, and lettuce rounds it out with mild, green freshness. It's like summer in a glass.

Ingredients

- 4 tomatoes
- 2 carrots
- 2 cucumbers
- 4 radishes
- 2 cups chopped romaine lettuce
- ½ lemon, peeled
- 1 stalk celery (optional)

Perfect For...

Getting your veggie fix on the go, a liquid lunch that actually fills you up, tricking yourself into healthier habits, or impressing friends who still think salad requires a bowl.

Side effects may include sudden cravings for more vegetables, an urge to start a garden, and a smug sense of superiority over salad-chewers. May not pair well with croutons. Do not attempt to add ranch.

ORANGE MOODS

Turn Up

When you need to get your roots in order and turn up your health game.

The Low Down

Who said you can't turn up with turnips? This root-tastic concoction proves that getting down with underground veggies can be a real party for your taste buds. Turnup is the drink that'll make you say, "Oh my gourd, I can't believe it's this good!" Time to get rooted in wellness.

Flavor Profile

An earthy symphony with sweet high notes. Sweet potatoes and carrots bring mellow sweetness, green apples add a tart twist, celery provides a fresh backdrop, and turnip greens offer a subtle peppery kick. Ginger ties it all together with a spicy zing that makes your taste buds dance."

Ingredients

- 1 small red potato or sweet potatoe
- 2 carrots
- 3 green apples
- 2 celery stalks
- 1/2 cup turnip greens (Substitute with 1/2 cup collard greens)
- 1 small turnip or a small rutabaga
- ½ inch ginger (optional)

Perfect For...

Grounding yourself in wholesome goodness, a pre-workout energy boost, a post-indulgence detox, or sneaking more veggies into your diet without anyone noticing.

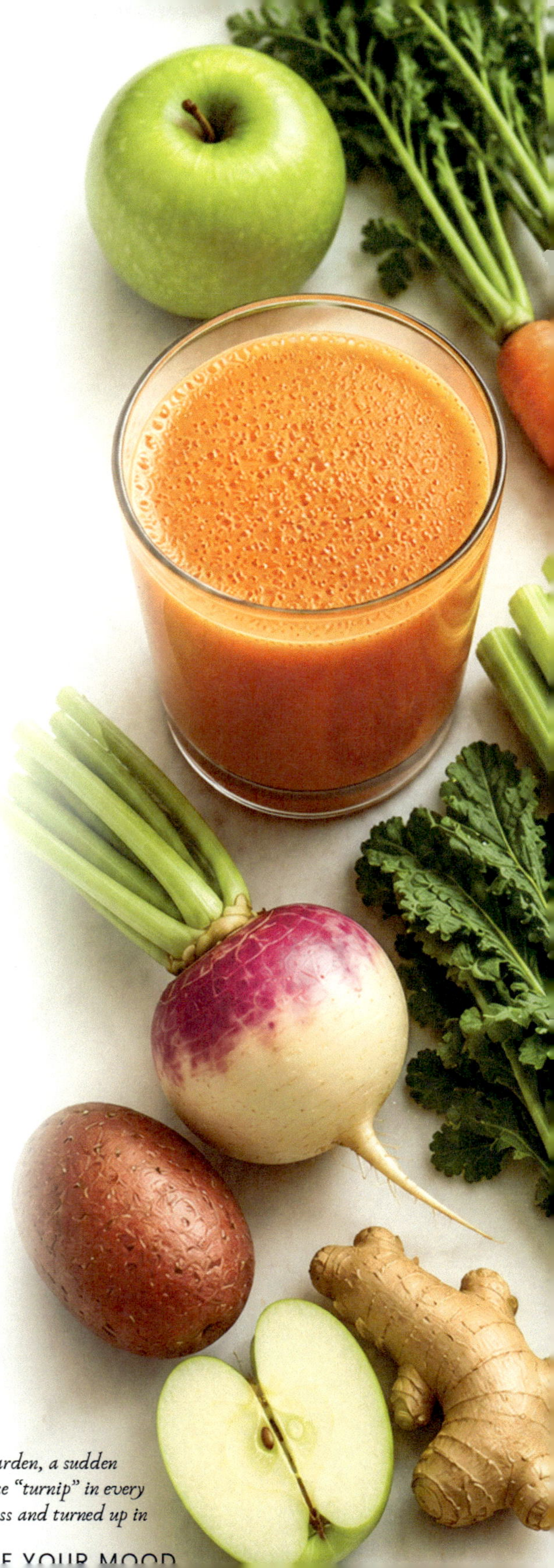

Side effects may include an inexplicable urge to garden, a sudden appreciation for root vegetables, and a desire to use "turnip" in every possible pun. May result in feeling rooted in wellness and turned up in life.

Unsure

When you don't
know how you
feel, but know you
need something.

The Low Down

Not every day comes with a clear mood. Sometimes you're just... here. Unsure is the "I don't know, you pick" of juices. Balanced, familiar, and impossible to get wrong. It's a safe place to land when you can't decide.

Flavor Profile

A little sweet, a little tart, a little earthy. Apple and orange keep it friendly, carrot grounds it, lemon brightens it, and ginger gives it just enough "I'm doing something good for myself" energy. It's the juice equivalent of a shrug that turns into a smile.

Ingredients

- 2 apples (any kind)
- 2 oranges
- 2 carrots
- 1 lemon
- Small piece of ginger

Perfect For...

When you can't pick a mood, don't trust your feelings yet, or want something that works without overthinking it.

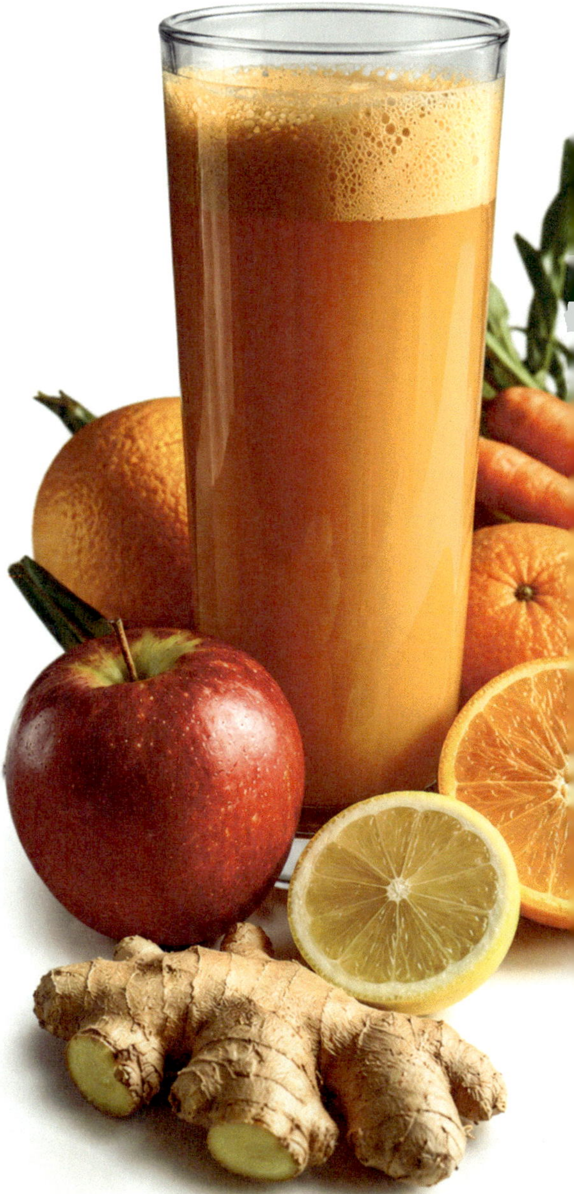

Side effects may include accidentally figuring out how you feel halfway through the glass. May lead to unplanned self-care and the realization that you're doing better than you thought.

Tasting a
perfectly ripe fruit
is like a little piece
of *sunshine.*

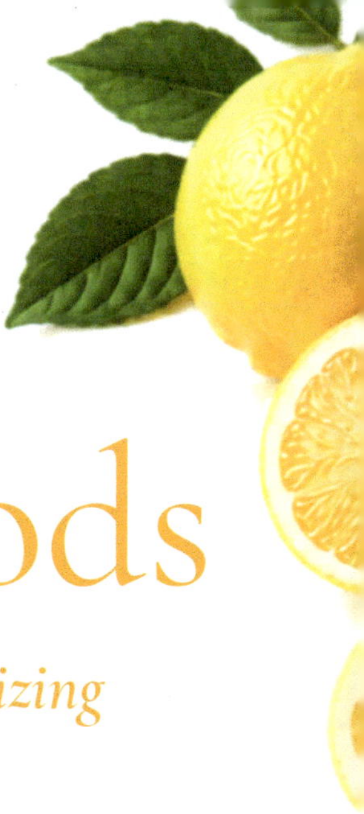

Yellow Moods

Bright, curious, and gently energizing

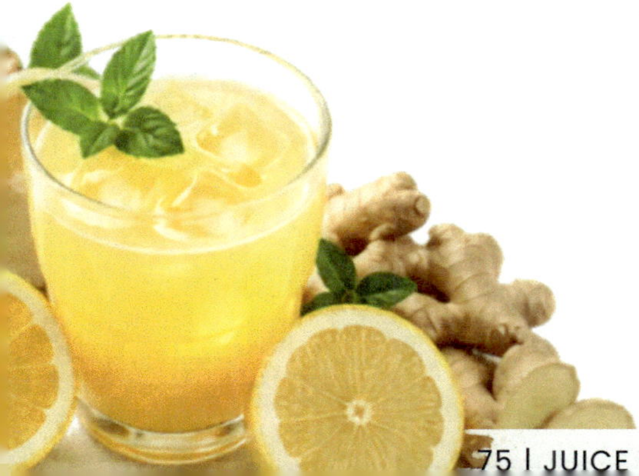

YELLOW MOODS

Cant Elope

When you are
committed to good taste
and running away
is not an option.

The Low Down

Say "I do" to this unconventional blend that's got more layers than a wedding cake!

Flavor Profile

Picture cantaloupe and potato as newlyweds, grapes in tow. Sweet, floral cantaloupe shines first, mellow potato follows, and grapes wrap it up. It's a tasty rom-com—playful, pleasant, and warm.

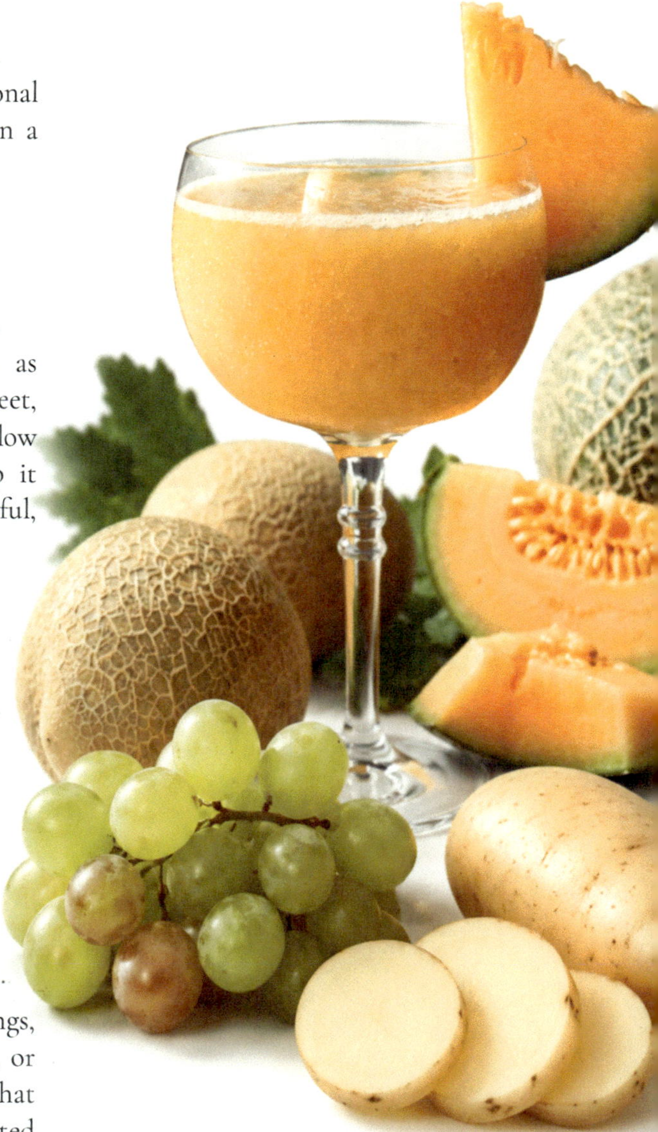

Ingredients

- 1 Cantaloupe
- 1 White Potato, peeled
- 2 cups of Green Grapes

Perfect For...

Sipping on lazy Sunday mornings, pre-gaming for wedding season, or anytime you need a reminder that sometimes the most unexpected combinations yield the sweetest results. It's also great for those moments when you're tempted to run away from your problems. This juice will convince you to stick around and juice it out!

Side effects may include an irresistible urge to propose to your blender, sudden cravings for honeymoon destinations, and the ability to commit to finishing the entire glass.

Lemon Pepper

When you need a bright
Reset with a little bite.

The Low Down

For the days when you need to snap out of it. Lemon Pepper is your reset button, bright, bold, and ready when you are.

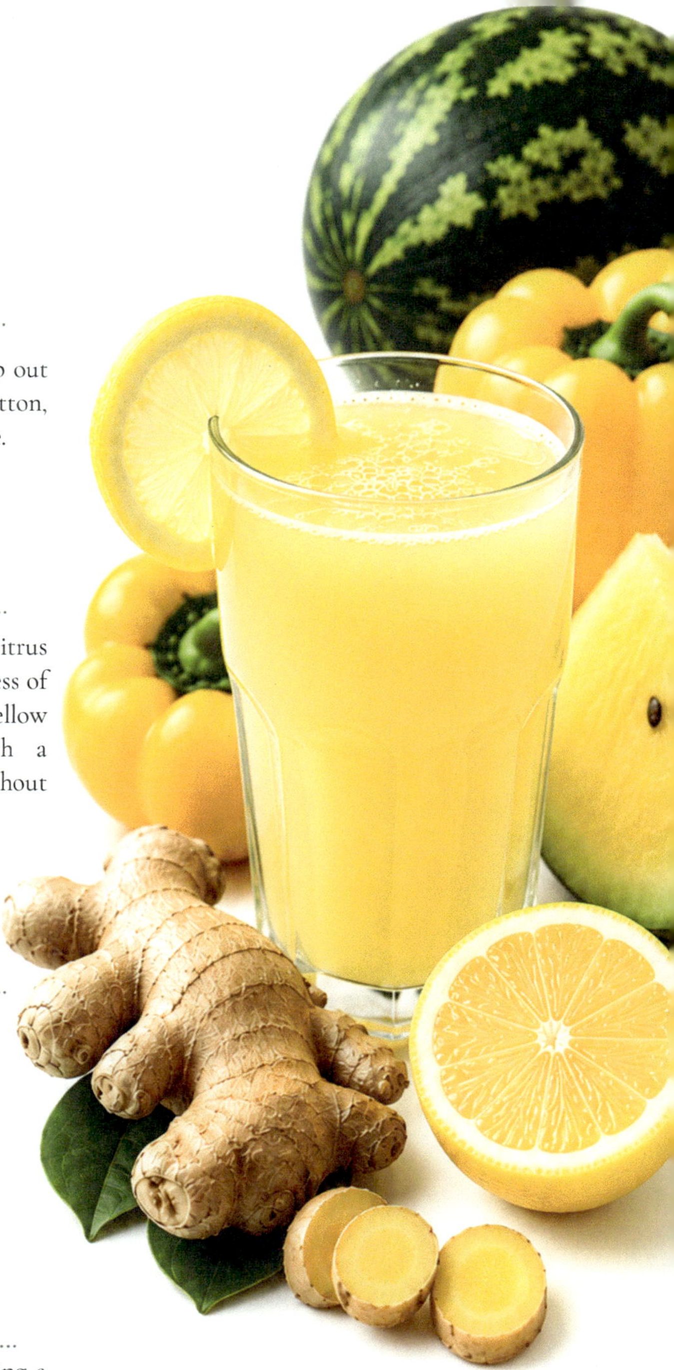

Flavor Profile

Zesty lemon leads with a clean citrus snap, balanced by the subtle sweetness of yellow bell pepper and yellow watermelon. Ginger finishes with a gentle warmth that lingers without overwhelming.

Ingredients

- 1 large lemon
- 1 yellow bell pepper
- 1 - inch fresh ginger
- 4 cups yellow watermelon (or honeydew melon)

Perfect For...

Shaking off sluggish energy, enjoying a midday reset without caffeine, or brightening up brunch and afternoon moments.

May cause heightened alertness, spontaneous optimism, and reduced tolerance for bland flavors. Side effects include seeing the bright side more often than planned.

YELLOW MOODS

Sweet Cheeks

When life feels
unhinged, but you're
still going.

The Low Down

Sweet Cheeks is sunshine with a mischievous streak. Juicy peaches, golden fruit, and tropical sweetness come together in a blend that feels like a compliment from a stranger and finding twenty dollars in an old jacket. Sweet, bright, and impossible not to like.

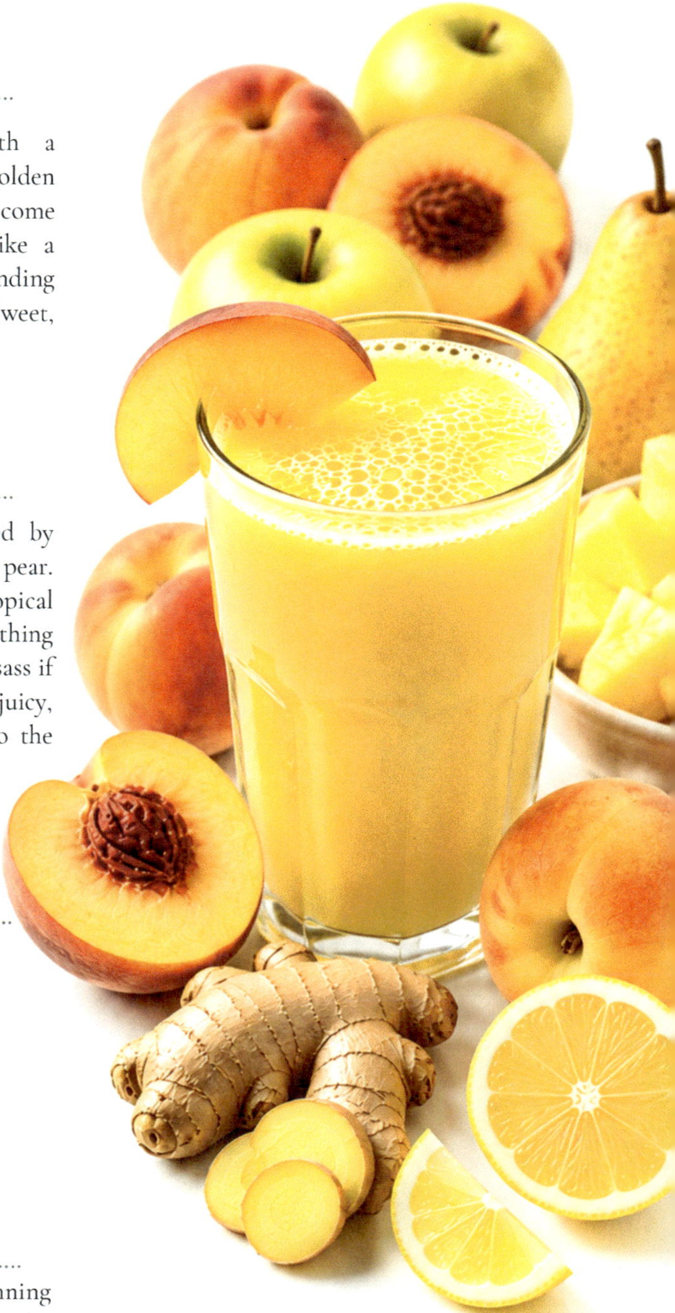

Flavor Profile

Soft peaches lead the way, backed by crisp golden apples and mellow pear. Pineapple adds a burst of tropical sweetness, lemon keeps everything balanced, and ginger brings a little sass if you choose to invite it. Smooth, juicy, and charming from the first sip to the last.

Ingredients

- 3 peaches
- 2 golden apples
- 1 cup pineapples
- 1 pear
- 1 lemon
- ½ inch ginger (optional)

Perfect For...

Busy days, spontaneous plans, running fashionably late, or anytime you need a little sweetness to keep moving forward.

May include unexpected confidence, excessive smiling, a spontaneous booty shake, and the belief that everything will work out just fine. You may also find yourself buying peaches without a plan.

Sometimes
you need to
step back
to see the
bigger picture.

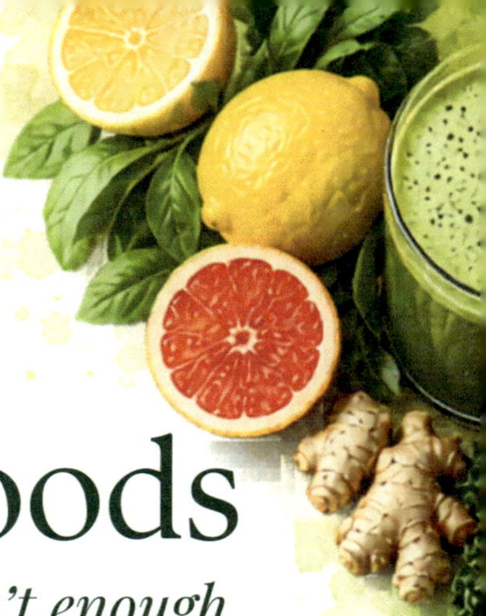

Mixed Moods

When one mood just isn't enough

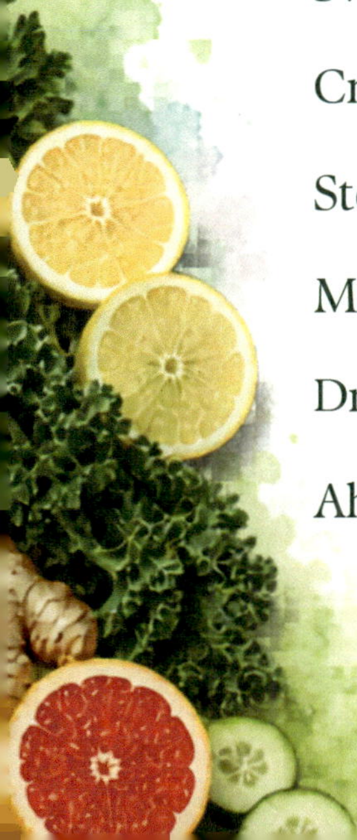

MIXED MOODS

Fearless Joy

When you need
courage AND
happiness in one glass.

Brave Soul + Chuckle

The Low Down

Courage with a grin. This blend lifts your spirits while giving you that zesty push to show up.

Flavor Profile

Bright lemon and cool cucumber meet sweet watermelon and cherry. Ginger adds a confident warmth.

Ingredients

- 1 lemon, peeled
- 1 cucumber, peeled
- 1 cup watermelon
- 1/2 cup cherries
- 1 cup red grapes
- 1/4 inch ginger (optional)

Perfect For...

Starting your day with confidence, celebrating small wins, or anytime you need to be brave AND enjoy it.

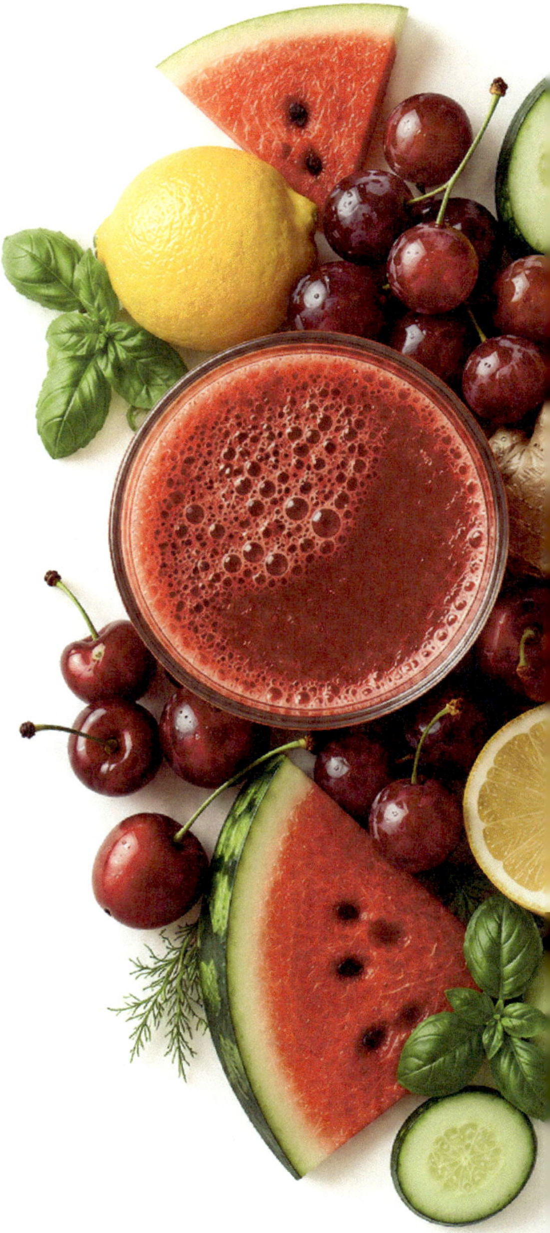

Side effects may include smiling at strangers, volunteering to go first, and laughing at your own jokes.

MIXED MOODS

Munday

When you're grumpy
but need to function.

Orange Sucker Punch + Bitter Grand

The Low Down

You didn't ask for Monday. Monday didn't ask for you. This juice gets you both through it.

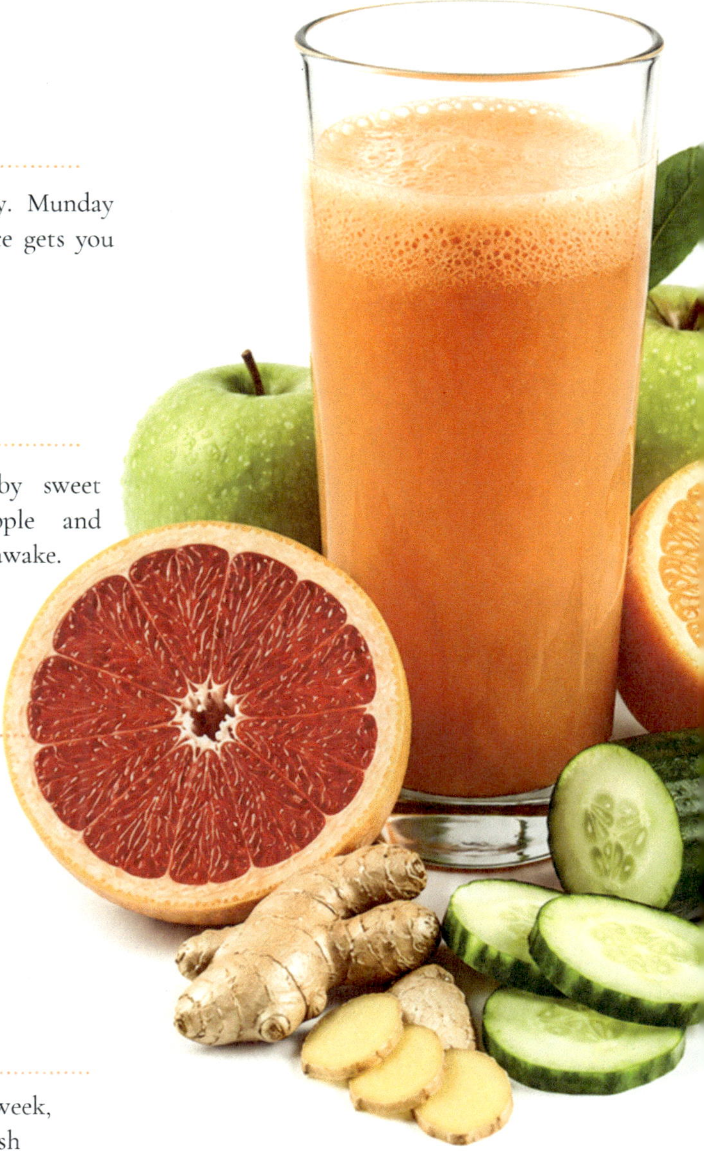

Flavor Profile

Tart grapefruit softened by sweet orange, grounded by apple and cucumber. Ginger kicks you awake.

Ingredients

- 1 grapefruit, peeled
- 2 green apples
- 2 oranges, peeled
- 1 cucumber peeled
- 1/2 inch ginger

Perfect For...

Surviving the start of the week, powering through a sluggish morning, or when coffee isn't cutting it.

Side effects may include tolerating your inbox, making eye contact before noon, and reluctant productivity.

MIXED MOODS

Quiet Storm

When feeling deep makes you thirsty

Deep + Thirsty

The Low Down

Calm on the outside. Fire on the inside. This juice is for the ones who are quiet but never weak. The ones brewing something powerful. You don't need to be loud to be a force.

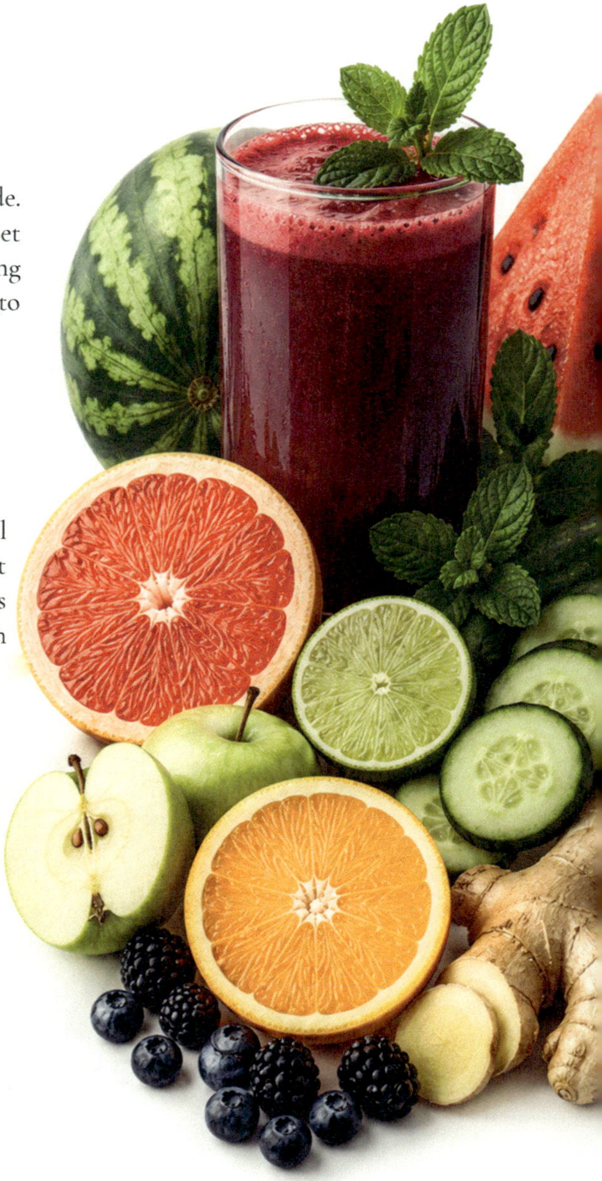

Flavor Profile

Deep berry richness meets cool cucumber and sweet watermelon. Mint refreshes, lime lifts, ginger sparks. It's calm with a current running through it.

Ingredients

- 1/2 cup blueberries
- 1/2 cup blackberries
- 1 cucumber
- 1 cup watermelon
- 4-5 mint leaves
- 1/2 lime, peeled
- 1/4 inch ginger (optional)
- 1/2 grapefruit, peeled

Perfect For...

When you're processing, plotting, or preparing to make a move. When calm is your superpower.

Side effects may include intense eye contact, quiet confidence, and the sudden realization that you've been underestimated.

MIXED MOODS

Fireside Flirt

When you feel cozy
and a little romantic.

Chilling Cherry + Winey

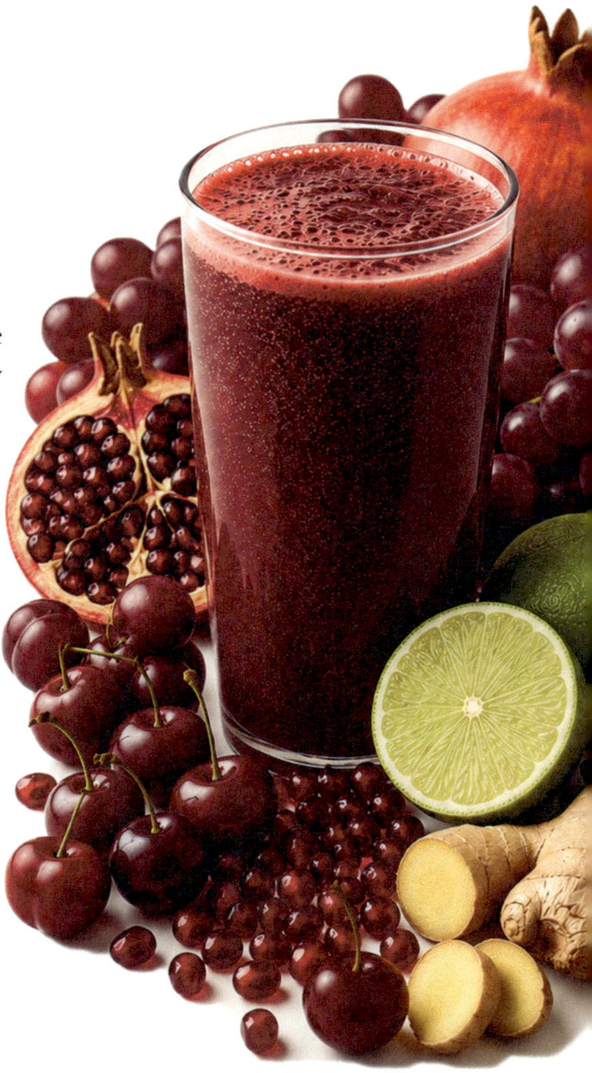

The Low Down

Warm, sweet, and just a little mysterious. Date night energy without leaving the house.

Flavor Profile

Lush cherries and deep pomegranate with grape sweetness. Lime brightens. Ginger warms.

Ingredients

- 2 cups cherries
- 2 cups red grapes
- 1/2 cup pomegranate seeds
- 1 lime, peeled
- 1/4 inch ginger
- ½ tsp cinnamon (optional)

Perfect For...

Date nights in, winding down with someone special, or treating yourself to something romantic, solo or not.

Side effects may include lingering eye contact, an unexplained urge to light candles, and texting someone 'hey' at 9pm. Consume responsibly

MIXED MOODS

Clean Slate

When you need a
reset, inside and out.

Tooted + Green Lemonade

The Low Down

We all need a reset sometimes. Clean Slate gives you a fresh start without the guilt. Just a simple way to clear out the old and make room for the new.

Flavor Profile

Earthy and bright with a cleansing finish. Brussels sprouts and celery bring that grounded, green energy, while tart green apple and bright lemon cut through with freshness. Cucumber adds smooth hydration, and ginger delivers a gentle kick that moves everything along. It tastes like you're doing something good for yourself and enjoying it

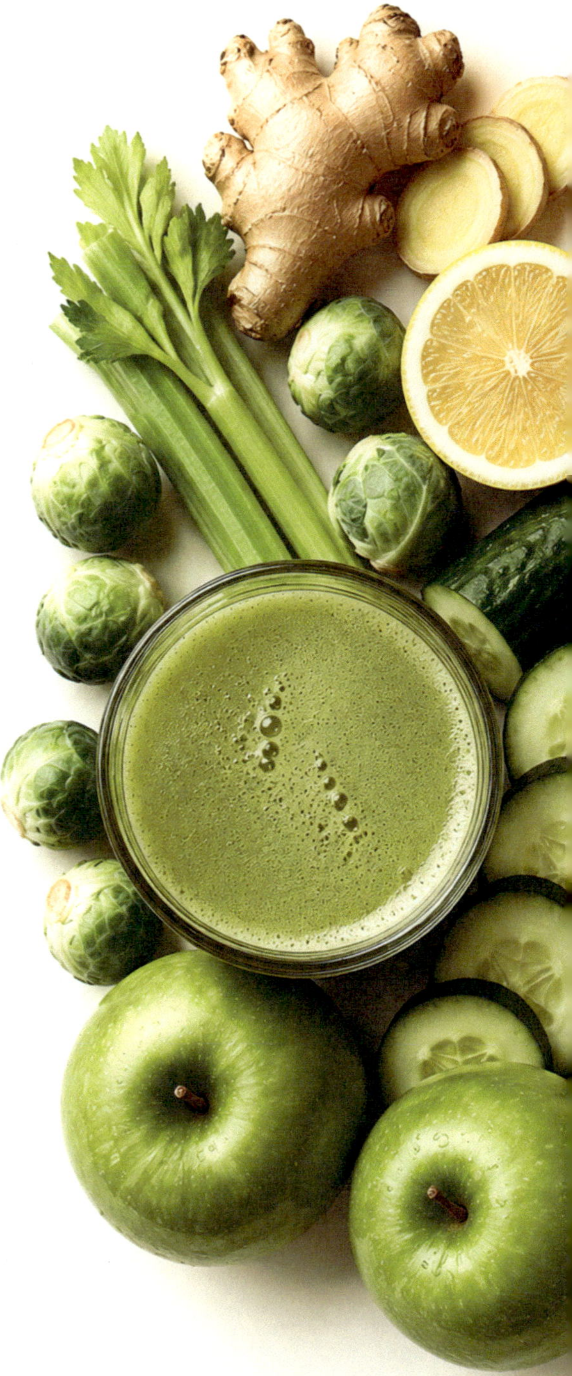

Ingredients

- 1 cup Brussels sprouts
- 2 celery stalks
- 2 green apples
- 1 lemon, peeled
- 1 cucumber
- 1/4 inch ginger

Perfect For...

Post-weekend resets, starting fresh after a rough patch, or when your body and mind both need a do-over.

Side effects may include sudden urges to organize, apologize, or start that thing you've been avoiding.

MIXED MOODS

Sweet Revenge

When you're salty, but choosing joy anyway

Salty + Thirsty

The Low Down

You're annoyed. But you're not letting it win. This combo lets you feel both and move on.

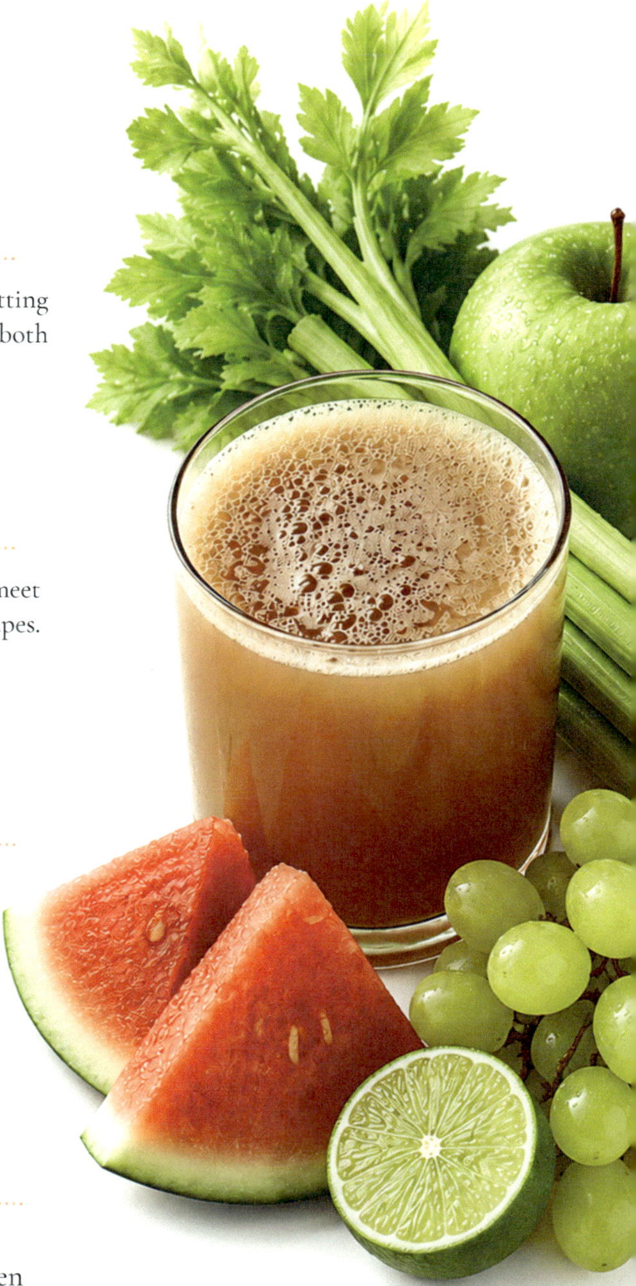

Flavor Profile

Mineral celery and tart apple meet sweet watermelon and juicy grapes. Salty start, sweet finish.

Ingredients

- 2 celery stalks
- 1 green apple
- 1 cup watermelon
- 1/2 cup green grapes
- 1/2 lime, peeled

Perfect For...

Getting over petty annoyances, choosing joy out of spite, or when you're salty but refusing to stay stuck there.

Side effects may include petty smiling, unbothered energy, and saying "I'm fine" and meaning it.

MIXED MOODS

Crown & Cozy

When you feel royal
AND relaxed

Purple Reign + Chilling Cherry

The Low Down

Who says you can't be royal and cozy? Crown & Cozy is for days when you want main-character energy without leaving the couch. It's comfy, it's playful, and it reminds you that you matter, even in sweats.

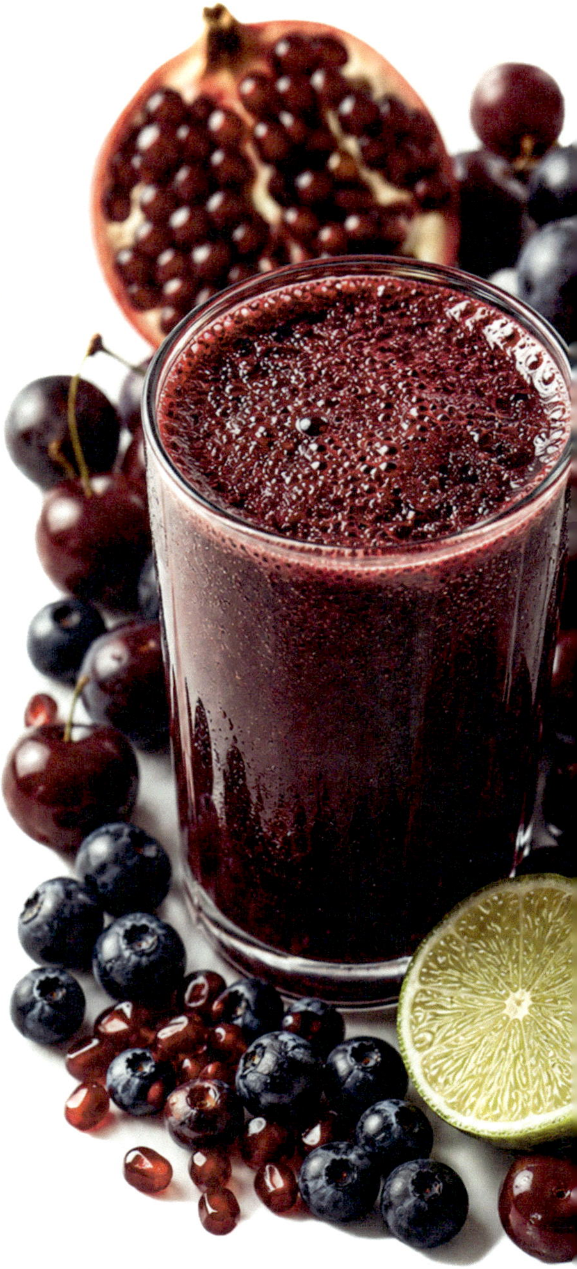

Flavor Profile

Deep, regal berries with sweet cherry warmth. Pomegranate adds jewel-toned richness. Lime keeps it bright.

Ingredients

- 1/2 cup black grapes
- 1 cup cherries
- 1/2 cup blueberries
- 1/4 cup pomegranate seeds
- 1/2 lime, peeled

Perfect For...

Feeling important without the pressure, or when you want to be the main character in your pajamas.

Side effects may include wearing a blanket like a cape, making royal decrees to your pets, and feeling quietly powerful.

MIXED MOODS

Steady

When you need
energy AND stability

Bloody Nose + Teacher's Pet

The Low Down

Steady powers you through busy days without the crash. It gives steady energy for big meetings, new projects, or anything that needs focus and strength.

Flavor Profile

Bold blood orange meets familiar apple sweetness. Grapes add depth. Lemon brightens. Cayenne whispers heat.

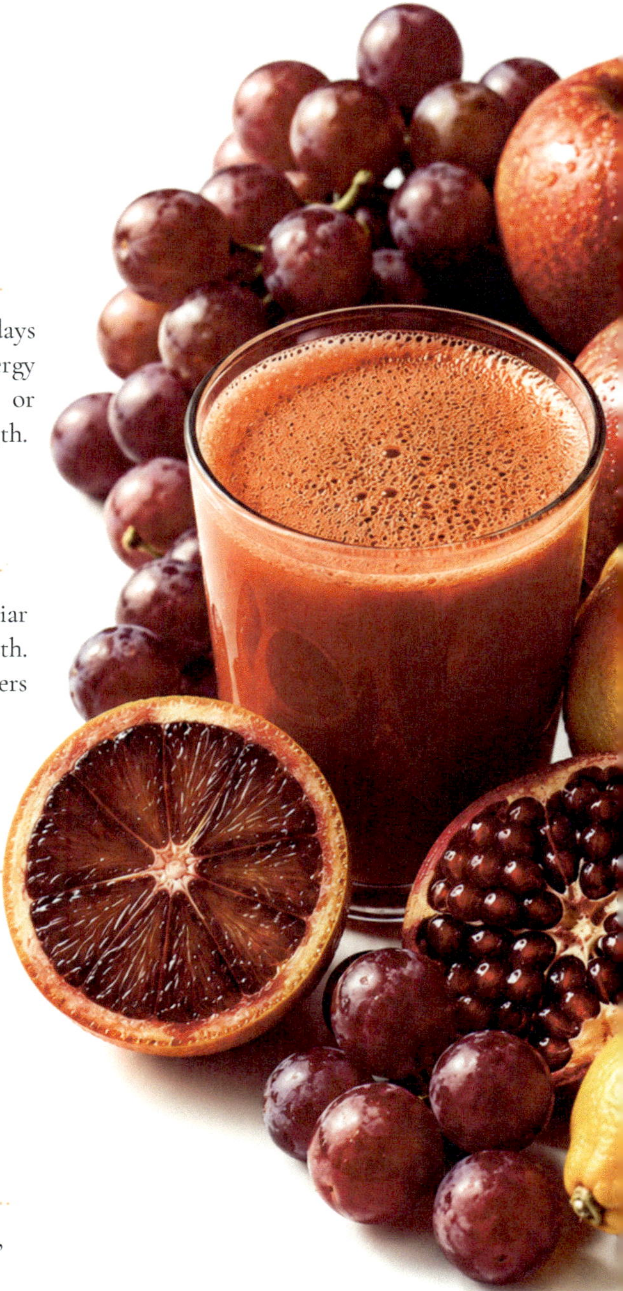

Ingredients

- 3 blood oranges, peeled
- 2 red apples
- 1 cup red grapes
- 1 lemon, peeled
- ½ tsp of cayenne (optional)

Perfect For...

Big presentations, job interviews, or any day you need to show up strong but stay grounded.

Side effects may include finishing your to-do list, raising your hand in meetings, and knowing your worth.

MIXED MOODS

Midnight Muse

When creativity meets clarity.

Night Owl + Green Lemonade

The Low Down

Midnight Muse is for when your brain won't quiet down, but you don't want it to. It's smooth, focused, and just stimulating enough to keep the ideas flowing without overwhelming you.

Flavor Profile

Deep blackberry mystery meets bright citrus clarity. Apple and cucumber keep it crisp. Ginger sparks the mind.

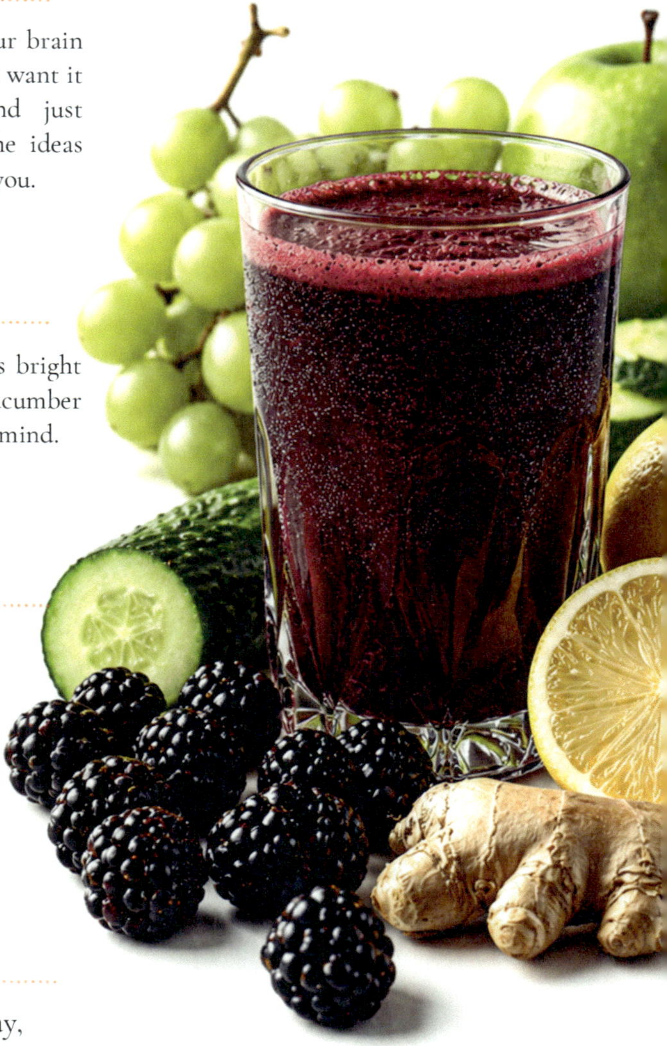

Ingredients

- 1 cup blackberries
- 1/2 cup green grapes
- 1 green apple
- 1/2 cucumber, peeled
- 1 lemon, peeled
- ¼ inch ginger

Perfect For...

Winding down after a long day, satisfying sweet cravings without the guilt, cozy evenings, or anytime you want a drink that feels like a hug.

Side effects may include filling notebooks, 3 am epiphanies, and saying "just one more idea.

MIXED MOODS

Dressed to Impress

When you want fancy
AND fresh

Tossed Salad + Winey

The Low Down

This isn't your average veggie juice. It's the one that shows up looking effortless but put-together. Crisp, bright, and a little bougie. You drink this when you want to feel like you have your life together—even if you don't.

Flavor Profile

Tomatoes bring tangy sweetness, cucumber keeps it cool, carrot adds earthy depth, and the grapes—red and black—make the whole thing feel fancy. Lemon ties the bow. It's a salad that showed up to the party in heels

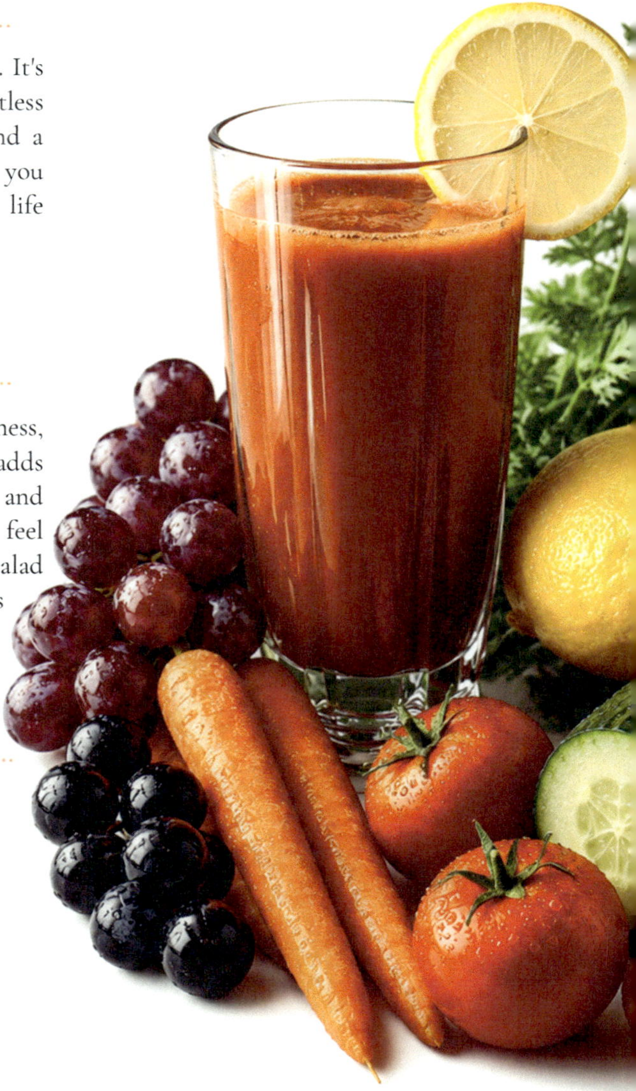

Ingredients

- 2 tomatoes
- 1 cucumber
- 1 carrot
- 1/2 cup red grapes
- 1/2 cup black grapes
- 1/2 lemon, peeled

Perfect For...

Brunch with friends, feeling fancy on a random Tuesday, or when you want to eat your veggies like they're expensive.

Side effects may include saying "darling" unironically, garnishing everything, and feeling effortlessly chic.

MIXED MOODS

Ahh, Finally

When you need relief
AND a reason to smile

Bloated and Chuckle

The Low Down

You know that moment when everything just... settles? Ahh, Finally that feeling in a glass. It's soothing, refreshing, and just playful enough to remind you not to take things too seriously. Light, easy, and exactly what you needed, even if you didn't know it yet.

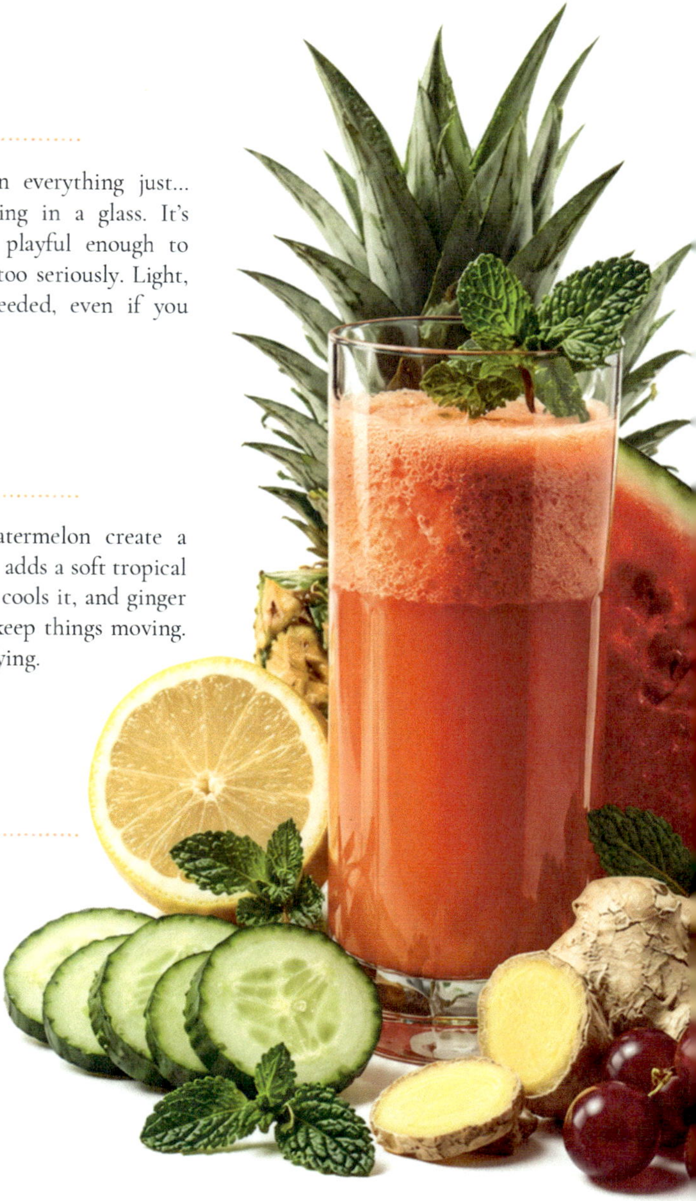

Flavor Profile

Cool cucumber and sweet watermelon create a refreshing base, while pineapple adds a soft tropical brightness. Lemon lifts it, mint cools it, and ginger brings just enough warmth to keep things moving. Smooth, light, and quietly satisfying.

Ingredients

- 1 cucumber
- 1 cup pineapple chunks
- 1 inch ginger
- 1/2 lemon, peeled
- A few mint leaves
- 2 cups watermelon
- 1 cup red grapes

Perfect For...

Post-meal relief, resetting your body and your mood, or when you just want to feel better without overthinking it.

Side effects may include Unbuttoning nothing, sighing dramatically (in a good way), and realizing everything's actually okay.

Thanks for *juicing with me.*

Before you go, here's a quick look at what's in your glass—and why it matters.

Fruits

What's in your glass?

Each fruit brings its own benefits, flavor, and mood.
Use this guide to mix, match, and sip with purpose.

Blackberries: Bold and grounding.
Packed with fiber and nutrients that support immunity and balance.

Blueberries: Small but powerful.
Brain-boosting and perfect for focus, clarity, and mental sharpness.

Cherries (Red & Black):
Deep and soothing.
Rich in antioxidants that help ease inflammation and support restful nights.

Cranberries: Tart and cleansing.
Support urinary health while giving your body a fresh reset.

Grapes (Red, Black, Concord, Green):
Sweet and heart-friendly—loaded with antioxidants and natural energy to keep you going.

Green Apples (Granny Smith):
Crisp and refreshing.
High in fiber and perfect for cutting through sweetness.

Kiwi: Tangy and revitalizing.
Packed with vitamin C and enzymes that aid digestion.

Pineapple: Tropical and soothing.
Contains enzymes that support digestion and ease bloating.

Pomegranate Seeds: Vibrant and powerful.
Support circulation and heart health with every sip.

Blood Oranges:
Bold citrus with depth.
Rich in rare antioxidants that boost immunity and flavor.

Cantaloupe:
Smooth and nourishing.
Supports hydration, heart health, and eye function.

Navel Oranges:
Classic and energizing.
Your go-to for vitamin C and a clean, bright taste.

Red Apples:
Balanced and naturally sweet.
Support immunity while rounding out bold flavors.

Raspberries:
Bright and fiber-rich.
Supports digestion while adding a tangy lift to your blend.

Strawberries:
Sweet and uplifting.
Rich in vitamin C to support glowing skin and immune health.

Watermelon:
Light, juicy, and refreshing.
Hydrating your body while helping you cool and reset.

Fun note: Ingredients support wellness, but they're not magic—your body still deserves water, sleep, and snacks. ♡

Hydrate | Rest | Nourish

Sources: USDA FoodData Central, NIH Office of Dietary Supplements,

Vegetables

What's in your glass?

Each vegetable brings its own benefits, flavor, and mood.
Use this guide to mix, match, and sip with purpose.

Beets: Deep and energizing—support blood flow and stamina while adding rich, earthy strength.

Broccoli: Strong and cleansing—supports detox pathways while delivering powerful nutrients.

Carrots: Sweet and steady—support eye health and immunity while naturally boosting flavor.

Collard Greens: Bold and nourishing—calcium-rich greens that support strength and detoxification.

Kale: Strong and grounding—nutrient-dense and supportive of overall balance and vitality.

Radishes: Sharp and awakening—add a peppery kick while supporting liver function and detox.

Spinach: Mild and versatile—rich in essential minerals while blending seamlessly into any juice.

Tomatoes: Juicy and heart-friendly—rich in antioxidants that support circulation and vitality.

White Potatoes: Neutral and grounding—provide a mild base and steady nourishment.

Bell Peppers: Bright and vibrant—packed with vitamin C to support skin, immunity, and clarity.

Brussels Sprouts: Hearty and grounding—rich in fiber and nutrients that support digestion and balance.

Celery: Light and replenishing—rich in natural electrolytes to support hydration and calm.

Cucumber: Cool and refreshing—hydrating and soothing, perfect for calming and balancing blends.

Purple Cabbage: Vibrant and protective—rich in antioxidants that support brain health and resilience.

Romaine Lettuce: Light and hydrating—a gentle green that supports digestion and easy blending.

Sweet Potato: Warm and sustaining—supports steady energy with fiber and natural sweetness.

Turnips & Turnip Greens: Earthy and revitalizing—support detox and bring depth to your blends.

Fun note: Ingredients support wellness, but they're not magic—your body still deserves water, sleep, and snacks.

Hydrate | Rest | Nourish

Sources: USDA FoodData Central, NIH Office of Dietary Supplements,

Citrus, Herbs & Spices

What's in your glass?

Each ingredient brings its own benefits, flavor, and mood. Use this guide to mix, match, and sip with purpose.

Cayenne Pepper:

Fiery and energizing—boosts circulation and metabolism with a bold, spicy kick.

Cinnamon:

Warm and comforting—helps balance blood sugar while adding cozy depth to your blends.

Ginger:

Spicy and invigorating—supports digestion, eases nausea, and adds a warming lift.

Mint:

Cool and refreshing—soothes digestion and brings a crisp, clean finish to any juice.

Lemons:

Bright and cleansing—rich in vitamin C and perfect for refreshing, detoxifying blends.

Rosemary:

Earthy and focused—supports memory and circulation with a subtle herbal note.

Limes:

Zesty and uplifting—add brightness while supporting absorption and overall vitality.

Turmeric:

Golden and grounding—known for its anti-inflammatory benefits and deep, nourishing warmth.

Fun note: Ingredients support wellness, but they're not magic—your body still deserves water, sleep, and snacks. ♡

Hydrate | Rest | Nourish

Sources: USDA FoodData Central, NIH Office of Dietary Supplements,

Find Your Mood Fast

Continued

Find Your Mood Fast

Continued

Find Your Mood Fast

Go ahead. Turn the page.

The *simple things* matter more than we think.

So, start with *what you have.* Build from there.

Grocery Checklist

All ingredients for the complete juice recipe book

Leafy Greens

- [ ] Kale
- [ ] Spinach
- [ ] Collard Greens
- [ ] Romaine Lettuce
- [ ] Turnip Greens

Other Vegetables

- [ ] Celery
- [ ] Cucumbers
- [ ] Brussels Sprouts
- [ ] Broccoli
- [ ] Radishes
- [ ] Tomatoes
- [ ] Carrots
- [ ] Orange Bell Pepper
- [ ] Yellow Bell Pepper

Root Vegetables

- [ ] Beets
- [ ] White Potatoes
- [ ] Sweet Potato
- [ ] Turnips

Apples

- [ ] Granny Smith Apples
- [ ] Red Apples
- [ ] Green Apples

Citrus

- [ ] Lemons Limes
- [ ] Blood Oranges
- [ ] Navel Oranges
- [ ] Oranges
- [ ] Grapefruit

Grapes

- [ ] Green Grapes
- [ ] Red Grapes
- [ ] Black Grapes
- [ ] Concord Grapes
- [ ] Dark Grapes

Cherries & Berries

- [ ] Red Cherries
- [ ] Black Cherries
- [ ] Blueberries
- [ ] Blackberries
- [ ] Strawberries
- [ ] Raspberries
- [ ] Cranberries

Melons & Tropical Fruits

- [ ] Watermelon
- [ ] Yellow Watermelon or Honeydew Melon
- [ ] Cantaloupe
- [ ] Pineapple
- [ ] Kiwi

Other Fruits

- [ ] Pear
- [ ] Pomegranate seeds
- [ ] Peaches

Herbs & Spices

- [ ] Fresh Ginger Root
- [ ] Fresh Mint Leaves
- [ ] Fresh Rosemary
- [ ] Cayenne Pepper
- [ ] Turmeric Powder
- [ ] Cinnamon

Tip: Check your pantry for spices before shopping — cayenne, cinnamon, and turmeric may already be there!

Sources: USDA FoodData Central, NIH Office of Dietary Supplements, National Center for Complementary and Integrative Health.

About Me

I started juicing in 2014, back when my four kids were younger, and my patience was shorter. I'm an Army veteran, a wife, a mom, and someone who believes a good juice can shift your whole day.

I'm still married to the love of my life, learning how to be kinder to myself (and him), and convinced that a good laugh fixes a lot of things—while sharing the house with two cats who think they run it.

Juice Your Mood isn't meant to be preachy or overly packed with nutritional data you'll forget five minutes later—the internet already does that. I just wanted to share how I see these juices: the colors, the moods, the vibes. If it motivates you to take care of yourself, even a little, that's enough for me.

Be kinder

than you were yesterday.

Take care

of yourself—one sip at a time.

Made in the USA
Las Vegas, NV
03 November 2026

57424182R00071